T0143249

Medicare Reform

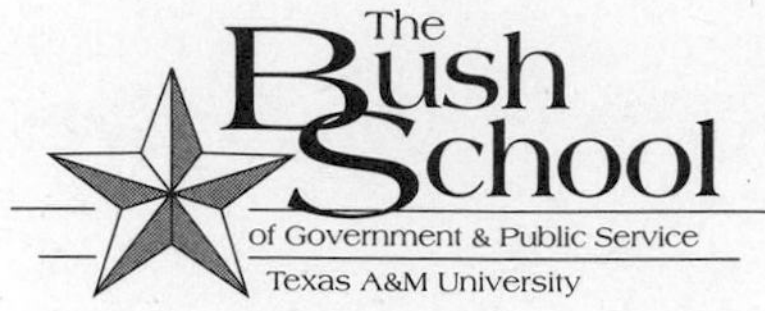

Volume I in the Bush School Series in the Economics of Public Policy

Edited by James M. Griffin

Medicare Reform: Issues and Answers

Edited by

Andrew J. Rettenmaier
Thomas R. Saving

The University of Chicago Press
Chicago & London

ANDREW J. RETTENMAIER is a research associate at the Private Enterprise Research Center, Texas A&M University.

THOMAS R. SAVING heads the Private Enterprise Research Center, Texas A&M University. A University Distinguished Professor of Economics at Texas A&M University, he also holds the Jeff Montgomery Professorship in Economics.

The University of Chicago Press, Chicago 60637
The University of Chicago Press, Ltd., London

08 07 06 05 04 03 02 01 00 99 1 2 3 4 5

ISBN: 0-226-71013-0 (cloth)

Library of Congress Cataloging-in-Publication Data

Medicare reform : issues and answers / edited by Andrew J. Rettenmaier and Thomas R. Saving.
p. cm.—(A volume in the Bush School series in the economics of public policy ; v. 1)
Collection of papers on Medicare reform from a 1998 conference.
ISBN 0-226-71013-0 (alk. paper)
1. Medicare Congresses. I. Rettenmaier, Andrew J. II. Saving, Thomas Robert, 1933– . III. Series: Bush School series in the economics of public policy ; v. 1.
RA412.3.M444 1999
368.4′26′00973—dc21 99-23001

♾ The paper used in this publication meets the minimum requirements of the American National Standard for Information Sciences—Permanence of Paper for Printed Library Materials, ANSI Z39.48—1992.

Contents

Foreword

When viewing our system of government from afar, many think it is primarily dominated by special interests. But the closer I look at the process and the more seriously I study it, the more convinced I become that in Washington, as in every other sphere of discussion, it is ideas that dominate, not special interests. One of the ideas on which there is a growing consensus is that something has to be done about entitlement programs for the elderly, especially Medicare. This book contains some new and important ideas on the subject of Medicare.

Almost no one in Congress fails to recognize the financial crisis arising from the explosive growth in the cost of Social Security and Medicare. It represents the largest financial crisis in the history of the country and most people know it. Every serious person has accepted the evidence produced by government and independent groups showing, at an absolute minimum, that the present value of the unfunded liability of Social Security and Medicare is at least twice the current measure of the outstanding public debt of the country. Under the best of circumstances, with the most enlightened reform program that can be instituted, the cost of paying off the unfunded liability of Social Security and Medicare is larger than the real expenditures on all the wars in the history of the country.

Now, what is the source of this problem? I believe the growing consensus among elected officials and those interested in public policy is that the source of the problem lies in financing these entitlements based on generational transfers. Nineteenth-century German chancellor Otto von Bismarck—in an emerging country with soaring population growth, relatively few older citizens, and a huge number of young workers coming into the labor market—conceived a political innovation that has affected virtually every country and now dominates the social programs of all Western countries. This political innovation was to recognize that you could substitute taxes on workers, yet unborn, for the age-old system of personal saving and investment to pay retirement benefits for current workers. Bismarck's innovation spread like wildfire across Europe, migrating to Australia in 1909, to the Americas in Chile in 1925, and to the United States in 1935 in the form of Social Security and in 1965 in the form of Medicare.

All these Bismarck systems have two problems. First, they create no wealth—no investment is made; no interest is earned—and so they are denied the benefit of what Albert Einstein called the most powerful force in the universe: the power of compound interest. Their ability to pay future benefits depends totally on the productivity of workers, the number of workers, and the willingness of those workers to bear the tax burden when the bills come due.

The second problem is that transfer payment systems are held hostage to demographics. In the latter half of this century, the expected life span has risen significantly; and since the end of the baby boom, the birth rate has collapsed. In the countries where these transfer payment systems are most entrenched, the birth rate has fallen furthest and fastest. The burden of the current system's cost will become oppressive even under the best of circumstances. Even if the economy is as strong as it is now every day for the next thirty years and with a fairly open policy of immigration supplying new workers, we will still require a payroll tax of roughly 30 percent to fund the current benefits of Social Security and Medicare. I do not think the devastating economic implications of a 30 percent payroll tax can be overstated.

I have reached the conclusion that we cannot solve this problem by cutting benefits and raising taxes. The level of cuts necessary to save the current Medicare and Social Security programs is not politically feasible, and the burden of taxes required to sustain the current system without program cuts is not economically sustainable in a competitive world.

So if you reach this conclusion, what is the good news? Well, I think there is a lot of good news. First of all, remember Einstein said that compound interest is the most powerful force in the universe. If a 22-year-old worker who is now paying 12.4 percent of his or her wages in Social Security taxes was allowed to put 3 percent of wages in a real investment (say 60 percent in stocks, 40 percent in bonds), that worker could generate over a working lifetime an asset that would fund his or her entire expected Social Security benefit. And with a reform of Medicare to bring the forces of competition to bear on medical purchases, the average 22-year-old worker, by setting aside 1.5 percent of wages—roughly one-half the current Medicare tax rate—could in a similar investment build an annuity that would buy the private equivalent of Medicare for the retirement years.

The final piece of glorious news is that such an investment-based system has already been tested, and it works. This is not a group of economics professors sitting around talking theoretically about what might be done—it has already been accomplished. Chile, a developing country once on the verge of bankruptcy, was able to restructure its debt-based transfer payment retirement system into a successful investment-based system. Chile has been using this system for seventeen years and is about to become the first country ever to achieve Karl Marx's dream of workers owning the means of production. However, unlike the Marxist system, individual workers in Chile really do own capital. A comparable transformation occurred in Australia under a Labour government. And, at least partially, a similar system was instituted in two-tier retirement benefits in Great Britain. Even Sweden, in 1998, began moving toward an investment-based system.

While an investment-based retirement system is taking root worldwide, the problems with retirement health care are more difficult but not insurmountable. Under Social Security, people are paid benefits based on what they have paid in; but under the Medicare system, people do not get different levels of coverage based on how much they have contributed. Medicare guarantees the same benefits to everyone. We are probably two or three years behind in looking at the impact of an investment-based Medicare system as compared to Social Security, but I think such a system can be made to work. This book provides a systematic discussion of the Medicare problem and explores an investment-based solution.

The problem with the transition to an investment-based Social Security system and Medicare system is not that the transition costs are big. The remarkable thing for anybody who has looked at any of these proposals is that it is cheaper over an extended period of time to get out of the current system and make a complete transition to a funded system than it is to stay in the current system. It is cheaper to fix it than it is to leave it broken, which is a revolutionary conclusion in the minds of many people. The challenge is a cash flow problem in the early years of the transition. If you are going to allow people to make real investments, they must do so at the same time they are paying for the benefits being collected by those under the old system. But as the television commercial says, "You can either pay me now, or pay me later," and investment-based Social Security and Medicare are the Fram oil filters of entitlement reform.

I believe that investment-based entitlement reform is going to happen, and I think it will happen because there is no feasible alternative. Some like the politics of having people dependent on the government, rather than on their own investments, and that will be the biggest hurdle to overcome. Opposition will come from people who prosper in the politics of the current system because of the political benefits they derive from public dependence on government. Stated more directly, the status quo will be defended not because it works economically but because it works politically.

Because, as Richard Weaver once said, "ideas have consequences," this book is important. It will not end the debate on Medicare, but it will begin it.

Senator Phil Gramm

Introduction

Andrew J. Rettenmaier
Thomas R. Saving

In the summer of 1965, the legislation establishing the Medicare program won congressional approval after years of consideration. In its original formulation, Medicare was to provide medical care insurance for the elderly population. Together with its sister program, Medicaid—which provides for the medical expenditures of the qualifying poor—they represent the Great Society's primary legacy. Without substantive changes, though, Medicare's legacy will turn into one of an ever-increasing tax burden on the working population. This dismal forecast arises from Medicare's financing arrangement, which makes the young responsible for the medical expenditures of the elderly. Historically, the growth in per capita expenditures has outpaced the growth in the young's average earnings. Combined with the demographic changes, which include longer periods of retirement and a bulge in the number of retirees, the implied tax rates that will be necessary in the near future will double. The funding problems are not unique to the Medicare program, though. The demographic changes contributing to Medicare's funding problems are shared with Social Security.

Because Medicare and Social Security support the elderly population, it is tempting to consider a uniform solution to their funding problems. However, the surface similarity that each program benefits the same population belies fundamental differences in what the programs

We are grateful to The Lynde and Harry Bradley Foundation for the funding that made our research and this conference possible. We also want to thank the members of the Private Enterprise Research Center staff for their assistance and perseverance during the planning stages and the actual conference. Our thanks go especially to Barbara Fisher, Susanne Lipinsky, and Lisa Riddick for their work preparing the final manuscripts.

do and in our society's requirements on them. Because health care has come to be viewed as a fundamental right, the quantity and quality of health care dispensed to the elderly bear less of a relationship to wealth status than does general retirement lifestyle. A second and equally important difference between Social Security and Medicare is the nature of the implied commitment to the elderly. Social Security fixes the total commitment and allows recipients to choose among alternative consumer goods to maximize individual satisfaction. Medicare, on the other hand, allows potentially unlimited expenditures so long as these expenditures take the form of what the system considers to be health care. These crucial differences in the two programs require that the solutions be related but different.

The sheer size of these elderly entitlements has always commanded considerable attention among policy makers and economists alike, but the fact that both programs are facing a trust fund crisis has brought renewed and serious scrutiny. Medicare and Social Security account for 35 percent of federal expenditures and over 7 percent of gross domestic product. By 2030 their collective share of gross domestic product is expected to reach almost 13 percent. At the present time, Social Security is receiving the bulk of the attention, even though Medicare's financial position is more precarious. Medicare spending now accounts for 2.65 percent of gross domestic product, and by 2030 its share is expected to rise to 5.85 percent. Further, the trust fund that is dedicated to the hospitalization portion of Medicare's two-part structure is expected to be depleted by 2008, three years prior to the retirement of the oldest of the baby boomers.

The approaching depletion of Medicare's hospitalization insurance trust fund has brought with it new urgency to finding a set of solutions to the program's problems. In the years leading up to Medicare's adoption, these potential funding problems were well-known in Congress and among the Social Security actuaries. The fact that even in the early 1960s the growth rate of medical expenditures was outpacing wage growth made congressional leaders leery of tying Medicare's finances to the Social Security program. But Medicare won passage in 1965, and, as congressional leaders had predicted, the payroll tax rate and tax base associated with funding hospitalization insurance have each been increased numerous times to keep pace with expenditure growth.

The early proponents of a federal program targeting the health care needs of the elderly argued that the market had failed to provide this group with affordable insurance. The elderly faced increasing medical costs on fixed incomes. At the time, the official poverty rate among the elderly was double that of the young. Proponents argued that by making the program universal, the poor would be covered and the nonpoor would not have the incentive to exhaust their savings to qualify. Further, they argued that universal coverage would insure the program would have general support. Interestingly, in the years leading up to its passage, most of the Medicare-type bills were limited to hospitalization insurance. It was not until after President Johnson was elected in a landslide in 1964 and Congress had its largest Democratic majority since the Roosevelt presidency that leaders in Congress who had opposed previous bills acquiesced; and eventually a bill that expanded coverage to include supplementary medical insurance was approved. The hospitalization insurance component of Medicare was and continues to be financed through payroll taxes. As part of the compromise legislation, the supplementary insurance was to be voluntary and financed through premium payments matched by general revenue funds. This two-part structure has persisted to today.

Often in a discussion of ways to reform the Medicare system, the focus is on how to curb expenditure growth or how to raise revenues, all in an attempt to balance the system's finances. However, at this point in the program's "life," it is worthwhile to consider more fundamental issues than just getting its finances in order. Federal programs tend to take on a life of their own and Medicare is no exception, as it has been expanded over the years far beyond its original scope. Benefits have been extended to individuals other than the elderly, the proportion of the costs of supplementary medical insurance borne by the federal government has risen, and Medicare's revenues have been tapped into to fund non–health care items such as graduate medical education.

The economic well-being of the elderly and the medical care marketplace have changed dramatically since the 1960s. The official poverty rate among the elderly has dropped from 28.5 percent in 1966 to 10.5 percent in 1997. Medicare's two-part structure has not evolved along with the development in the broader health insurance market. After thirty-four years, the time is ripe to reevaluate Medicare's basic structure and financing. The nature of Medicare's transfer payment financing combined with the imminent surge in the elderly population represented by the retirement of the baby boomers bind generations together such that future generations of workers will face substantial commitments to the retired population. Using the Trustee's 1998 estimates, the total unfunded commitments—expressed as the present value of the difference between projected revenues and expenditures—is $8.9 trillion, or 233 percent of the current national debt. The changing wealth status of the elderly and the structure of the medical market in which they receive services, as well as the looming liability, call for restructuring the system.

In a conference hosted by the Private Enterprise Research Center and the Bush School of Government and Public Service in conjunction with the Department of Economics at Texas A&M University, participants examined the core issues in the present Medicare reform debate and the answers being offered. This volume represents the collection of papers presented during the 3 April 1998 conference. The authors present quite divergent views on their interpretation of the issues facing Medicare and on the policy changes being suggested. Their views capture the spirit of many of the reforms being considered and provide the intellectual muscle behind those ideas. As a whole, their comments define the state of the current debate and delve into the issues that must be addressed if the system is to be fundamentally changed.

The fundamental issues can be divided between those pertaining to the intergenerational nature of Medicare's financing and those pertaining to perceived market failures. Medicare in its current form is financed on a pay-as-you-go basis, in that current benefits are paid out of contemporaneous tax revenues. The components on the revenue side of the pay-as-you-go accounting identity are the tax rate times aggregate earnings, where aggregate earnings are the product of average earnings and the number of workers. For the system's finances to balance, these revenues must equal the system's expenditures, which are the product of average benefits and the number of beneficiaries. The required tax rate is equal to the product of two critical ratios: the average benefit to average income ratio and the number of retirees to number of workers ratio. The greater the ratio of average benefits to average income, the greater the tax rate must be to balance the Medicare budget. Also, the greater the number of retirees relative to the number of workers, the greater the tax rate required for balancing the Medicare budget.

Once this fundamental accounting is understood, the source of the current Medicare crisis becomes clear. The past decade has seen a rapid increase in both of the critical ratios. Moreover, forecasts of future health care costs suggest that further increases in the ratio of average benefits to average income can be expected. Even worse, however, is the demographic reality that the pending retirement of the baby boom generation will significantly increase the ratio of beneficiaries to workers, the effect of which will be exacerbated by the expected further reductions in the fertility rate. Thus, the combination of an increasing benefits to earnings ratio and an increasing beneficiaries to workers ratio will place an impossible burden on the current pay-as-you-go system of Medicare finance. Since income cannot be directly influenced by policy, any solution to the Medicare crisis must in the end affect the two critical ratios by changing the level of benefits, the number of beneficiaries, or the number of workers.

Pay-as-you-go financing of intergenerational transfers is common across the globe, though the wisdom of such financing is being reconsidered in a growing number of countries. If Medicare's problems are to be seriously dealt with, its current financing arrangement must not be sacrosanct. Transfers between generations financed on a pay-as-you-go basis bind successive generations together in a contract that was not agreed upon by both parties. Over the first thirty-four years of the program, workers have borne much of the medical expenditure risk associated with paying Medicare benefits; and if the financing is left unchanged, they will bear the population size risk as well. There are alternatives to the current financing arrangement. One is to keep the current pay-as-you-go financing and limit taxes. This solution would shift the medical expenditures risk and/or the generation size risk toward beneficiaries and away from workers, by allowing average benefits to adjust to tax revenues. Another alternative is to move away from the current intergenerational compact—which relies on taxing the working generation to provide the primary source of funds for the retired generation's health care expenditures—to a system of financing retirees' health care expenditures through the accumulation of capital while a generation is in its youth, followed by the sale of the capital in its retirement.

Any solution to Medicare's financing problems must address the argument that reliance on an entirely private health care market may not provide adequate levels of health care for the elderly. There are several categories of the alleged market failure. The first suggests that in the absence of Medicare, the level of health care purchased by the elderly would be too low. Such a situation can arise if the societal benefits are not limited to individuals who directly consume medical care. If the young as a group care about the elderly's health care consumption, then government intervention can solve the free-rider problem. Taxes on the young can be collected and distributed to the elderly in such a way that the optimal level of medical care is consumed. However, the intervention need not be in the form of a universal subsidy but can be limited to cases in which the privately purchased level of care is deemed to be insufficient. If the inadequacy of care is inversely related to income, a means-tested subsidy can be justified.

Often, though, the inadequate care is also related to the health status of an elderly individual. The most common justification for the Medicare system is that it addresses the joint problems that arise from poverty and health status. It is argued that in the absence of Medicare, the ill could not and the poor would not buy insurance. As a society, we have decided that the elderly will receive some minimum level of care. In practice, the care is meted out to the elderly through their use of a government-sponsored insurance policy. Another, apparently implicit, goal of the program is to provide a uniform level of insurance to the elderly. The mutual goals of equal access and equal insurance coverage are accomplished through a universal and identical insurance policy.

Even if an identical universal health insurance subsidy for the elderly persists in the wake of the mounting financial strains on the system, it remains unclear to many that a federal entity need be the insurer. Recent changes to the system have allowed private insurers to enter the Medicare market in greater numbers and in changing capacities. In addition to health maintenance organizations (HMOs), Medicare beneficiaries will soon have the opportunity to choose among private fee-for-service (PFFS) plans, preferred provider organizations (PPOs), and provider-sponsored organizations (PSOs). Beginning in 1999, medical savings accounts (MSAs) will be an option for about 1 percent of Medicare's beneficiaries as a demonstration project that is currently scheduled to end in 2003. All of these private-sector options come with the promise of controlling per capita expenditure growth. Further changes in the market could open the door for innovative insurance contracts that can potentially overcome adverse selection on the part of beneficiaries and screening on the part of market entrants.

The fairness of the intergenerational contract and the issues in the health care market in general are not simple topics to tackle, but they must be thoroughly considered in a debate on reforming a system with over 36 million beneficiaries. In one way or another, each chapter in this volume touches on these issues. They do so by exploring the universal nature of the program, the degree to which it redistributes between and within generations, the benefits and costs of public versus private intervention, and issues unique to health care markets for the elderly. Because the full effect of the baby boomers' transition from taxpayers to benefit recipients is looming on the horizon, those who offer corrective action seem to agree that reform today is preferred to reform later. The papers and comments appear in their order of presentation with a final chapter by the editors. As we discuss each chapter, we will emphasize its place in the general solution space of average benefit levels, numbers of beneficiaries, and numbers of workers.

Victor R. Fuchs, in "'Provide, Provide': The Economics of Aging," explores the joint economic issues of increased health care utilization and decreased earning power associated with aging. Fuchs covers the gamut of the solution space, suggesting policy changes that increase the incentives for the elderly population to work (thus increasing the working population), which will allow them to pay a greater share of their medical care expenses (thus reducing benefits and number of beneficiaries). But the paper does much more than just suggest solutions to the current crisis; it also investigates aspects of the aging population that have heretofore been neglected.

Fuchs analyzes the effect of the changing patterns of health care utilization on the level of income inequality that exists among the elderly. He begins by pointing out that if health care expenditures continue on their historical path, by 2020 elderly health care expenditures will consume one-tenth of the nation's output. Fuchs suggests that most of the growth in overall health care expenditures by the elderly is not a result of changing demographics or prices but a change in per capita utilization. He shows that Social Security and Medicare reduce income inequality among the elderly below the degree of inequality that exists among the young.

Fuchs points out that the elderly's health care consumption is a public policy issue because taxpayers, rather than the elderly, are responsible for a majority of the expense. Because the government can affect the benefits ratio and the rate of per capita benefits growth, how it behaves influences technological advances. What the government pays for in terms of covered procedures and in terms of subsidies greatly influences the path of expenditure growth. Fuchs suggests that paying for the growth, aside from higher levels of intergenerational transfers, can be partially accomplished through changing government policies that produce disincentives for elderly labor force participation—namely, reducing or eliminating the high implicit tax rates facing the elderly. Such policy changes would increase the number of workers and allow the elderly to pay for more of their health care expenditures, thereby simultaneously decreasing the benefits to income ratio and the beneficiaries to workers ratio. Even with no change in the Medicare system, Fuchs emphasizes that increased savings by the elderly, either voluntary or mandatory, are the most important implication of his health expenditures forecasts.

In "Medicare Choice: Good, Bad, or It All Depends," Henry J. Aaron primarily addresses the provisions of the Balanced Budget Act of 1997 that allow Medicare beneficiaries expanded choice of their insurer. Since expanded choice has the potential of reducing benefit expenses, Aaron's chapter is suggestive of the first item in the solution space. Aaron, however, also incorporates an expansion of Medicare coverage that may contribute toward a net increase in benefits.

In the course of his discussion, Aaron comments on issues ranging from the rationality of economic agents, to paternalism, to adverse selection—all of which require consideration in a debate about choice in health care markets. Aaron poses three questions at the outset: Is more choice a good thing? Will the expansion of choice work to benefit patients? Will the reforms in the Balanced Budget Act pave the way for further modification of the program in the years leading up to the baby boomers' retirement? Aaron argues that these reforms will hinder further reforms because they will raise the cost of implementing a package he prefers—one with a standardized but expanded set of benefits.

To develop his case, Aaron suggests that choice in general is a good thing, but that limiting choice in the health care market may improve welfare. He argues that the complexity of possible health care insurance contracts may be beyond customers' abilities to choose among them. Secondly, in the health insurance market, no equilibrium may exist because insurers cannot effectively discriminate among customers with differing risks and preferences due to asymmetric information. As a result, welfare may be higher if insurance options are limited to a single plan, possibly with mandatory participation. Thirdly, even if the insurance market produces stable outcomes, these outcomes may be inferior to universal coverage. Additionally, individuals' choices may be time inconsistent, and, as a result, annual shifts between policies may not be optimal. Aaron also comes to the defense of paternalism in that it reflects an accurate judgment that private decisions produce consequences no compassionate society will tolerate.

In light of these perceived failures resulting from choice in the health insurance market, Aaron advocates the establishment of a uniform and liberalized coverage. Uniformity addresses the issues of risk selection and his contention that intelligent comparison of the costs of plans is impossible when the benefit packages differ. While noting that the expanded coverage and uniformity will increase the government's costs, Aaron suggests that these reforms would lower total medical spending adjusted for quality.

Mark V. Pauly's contribution—"Should Medicare Be Less Generous to Higher-Income Beneficiaries?"—addresses, both theoretically and empirically, the issue of means-testing elderly entitlements. The conclusions in this chapter fit into the reducing beneficiaries element of the solution space. In effect, by means-testing eligibility for Medicare benefits, Pauly transfers part of the retired population from pay-as-you-go financing to prepaid financing, thus reducing the apparent tax burden.

Pauly outlines a variety of related reforms of Medicare. First, since being old is no longer synonymous with being poor, Medicare generosity can be tied inversely to income. He bases his conclusion on the premise that the relatively wealthy will consume at least socially adequate levels of care without subsidies, and therefore subsidies are not required. Pauly argues further that by moving toward a program in which higher-income or wealthier beneficiaries receive smaller transfers, we will improve both equity and efficiency. His argument is persuasive if one assumes that the only reason for the Medicare elderly entitlement is to ensure that the elderly consume an "adequate" quantity of health care. Further, the way in which Medigap supplements interact with Medicare payments increases the inefficiencies by encouraging excessive use of the health care system.

Pauly suggests a partial solution to Medicare's financing crisis that encompasses reducing the expected growth in the benefits income ratio by shifting quality-of-care risk to beneficiaries. In particular, Pauly advises that Medicare should in the future only cover access to roughly 1998 quality, rather than state-of-the-art 2020, medicine. His position points to the intergenerational nature of the transfer payments embodied in Medicare benefits. He argues that in the future there needn't be a commitment to provide a higher-quality level than exists today for future Medicare beneficiaries in general and, for reasons cited above, to the well-to-do beneficiaries in particular. The normative questions he raises are issues of how much of the improvements in health care are owed to future cohorts of the elderly.

The unique characteristics of Pauly's proposal include cutting the amount of Medicare payments made on behalf of beneficiaries, on a basis that is positively related to income or wealth. He also suggests that under the pay-as-you-go financing arrangement, the current tax rates on wages are sufficient to maintain future benefits at the current levels in real terms, even with the coming demographic changes—which raises once again the question of who should pay for any future technological advancements: beneficiaries or taxpayers? Pauly concludes by arguing that Medicare should be blended more smoothly with other social programs, the end goal being an integrated package of age-related taxes and subsidies.

Marilyn Moon, in "The Limits of Economic Incentives," comments on the papers by Fuchs, Aaron, and Pauly. Moon's emphasis is on expanding the Medicare reform discussion beyond economics. She expresses her concerns that the private sector has never served the elderly and disabled populations well, and she favors continued government provision. She argues that a narrow definition of efficiency, which only accounts for market economic costs, is not appropriate in the health care market. Moon closes by suggesting that distributional issues between generations and consumers' desires for apparently inefficient levels of health care services are best handled in a broader context than one that rests solely on the criteria of economic efficiency.

Frank A. Sloan and Donald H. Taylor Jr.'s "Does Ownership Affect the Cost of Medicare?" examines the difference in the expenses that accrue to Medicare from for-profit and not-for-profit hospitals. This chapter analyzes the potential impact of institutional changes on benefit levels and thus fits into the benefits dimension of the solution space. In particular, they explore whether the rapid growth of the for-profit hospital sector has played a significant role in the rapid growth of benefits per capita.

Sloan and Taylor investigate the relative performance of nonprofit, for-profit, and public hospitals. Medicare's payments to hospitals differ based on the hospital's location, whether or not the hospital is a teaching institution, and the degree to which the hospital treats low-income patients. The questions addressed are how do ownership and teaching status affect Medicare payments and health outcomes?

The authors use panel data on individuals who were admitted to hospitals with a serious diagnosis. They then track the costs accruing to Medicare and the outcomes associated with the patients' treatments. Outcomes are measured in terms of mortality, rehospitalization, living arrangements, and functionality. They find evidence that beneficiaries admitted to for-profit hospitals are more costly than those admitted to public hospitals and less costly than those admitted to major teaching hospitals. Relative to patients admitted to nonprofit/nonteaching and minor teaching hospitals, those admitted to for-profit hospitals did not generate statistically significantly greater Medicare costs. Survival rates of patients admitted to major teaching hospitals were better than survival rates at other hospitals, but there were no significant differences between the outcomes generated at for-profit hospitals and the other hospital categories. By and large, performance of the different types of hospitals is found to be very similar, with major teaching hospitals being more expensive but providing better-quality care. Sloan and Taylor conclude that the implication for Medicare is that differences in cost and quality between nonteaching for-profits and nonprofits are on the whole minimal; thus, the cases of Medicare fraud and abuse in the for-profit sector that have received recent media attention are isolated cases and cannot be generalized to all for-profits.

In "What Does Medicare Spending Buy Us?" David M. Cutler tackles the topic of medical expenditure growth. Cutler's work deals with the benefits component of the solution space. He investigates the cause of the rapid growth of benefits and suggests incentive changes that may control this growth.

Cutler decomposes medical care expenditures into price, quantity, and quality effects. He uses the case of heart disease interventions to show how real expenditures have risen at the same time that real prices for each component of the set of four treatments have either declined or risen modestly. The increase in total expenditures is accounted for by a shift toward the use of more-intensive treatments. Cutler quantifies the costs and the benefits of Medicare by comparing real spending to a monetized measure of increased longevity and enhanced quality of life. He suggests that even if only one-quarter of the estimated benefits were the result of Medicare spending, the additional spending would be worth it. He hastens to say that although the increased spending is worth it, an appreciable fraction of Medicare spending and health care expenditures in general produce little in the way of health benefits. He attributes the purchase of services that yield low additional values to the incentives built into the health care system. Given that insured individuals pay little for additional services, they have the incentive to demand care that yields little additional value.

In light of his conclusions that Medicare spending has been worthwhile but that it also wastes resources, Cutler offers several reform suggestions. First, he does not recommend that Medicare be put on a budget, because it is not certain how much should be spent. A budget may produce the wrong incentives and as a result would not address the more fundamental issues. Cutler utilizes his analysis of medical care prices and utilization to argue that historical attempts at controlling Medicare's cost by reducing payment rates have not been and are not likely to be long-run solutions. Such solutions focus on prices, when, in reality, expenditure growth has come in the form of increased quantity. His third point is that shifting more of the health care costs to Medicare beneficiaries is a good policy but must be part of a broader solution that also addresses the issue of inappropriate care. Cutler's final suggestion deals with incentives within the Medicare system. The system Cutler advocates is a choice-based system. The choice-based system would have many of the attributes of current employer health programs, in which beneficiaries would choose from a menu of options and Medicare would contribute a fixed amount. Cutler points out that such a system for Medicare may require substantial regulation on insurers, such as a requirement to take all applicants, allowing for renewal regardless of existing conditions, and uniform pricing. However, he sees a workable system of marketplace incentives as the highest priority issue in the Medicare reform debate.

Jagadeesh Gokhale and Laurence J. Kotlikoff use their generational accounting methodology in "Medicare from the Perspective of Generational Accounting" to identify the Medicare cuts that would be required to balance the generational accounts under the status quo and several alternative Medicare systems. Their work emphasizes the impact of a generation size shock, such as the baby boom generation, on the tax rates required to finance any benefits-income ratio. While they do not suggest policies that will solve the problem, they estimate the size of the problem with which any suggested solution must cope.

Gokhale and Kotlikoff identify the degree to which current and future generations suffer as the result of participation in programs that transfer resources from the young to the old. Generational accounting identifies the net tax payments—lifetime taxes paid less lifetime benefits received—for each existing age group and for future generations. Ideally, at birth each new generation would be in a situation where it could expect to receive benefits equal to the taxes it is expected to pay. Because of the significant unfunded liability embodied in the Medicare program, current newborns can expect to pay federal taxes far in excess of any expected federal benefits.

The chapter also identifies the net tax payments of current and future generations in the United States and around the world. The authors decompose the accounts for male and female cohorts in the United States by type of tax and type of benefit. They estimate the reduction in promised Medicare benefits required to make the lifetime net tax rates of newborns and future generations equal, a situation referred to as establishing generational balance. Gokhale and Kotlikoff estimate that Medicare benefits would have to be cut 68 percent in 1998 to bring the generational accounts into balance; and if reform is postponed until 2003, benefits would have to be permanently cut by 78 percent. If reform is delayed until 2016, just five years into the retirement of the oldest group of baby boomers, even the complete elimination of the program would not produce generational balance!

Kevin M. Murphy, in "Asking the Right Questions in the Medicare Reform Debate," comments on the papers by Sloan and Taylor, Cutler, and Gokhale and Kotlikoff. Murphy argues that one must be careful to ask the right question if one expects the answer to be of value. Any discussion of Medicare must make the distinction between Medicare and medical care. Wanting to reform the first does not imply reforming the second. Murphy emphasizes that a critical consideration in deciding how much care the elderly ultimately receive is who is paying the bill and how the bill is paid. Further, he suggests that part of the solution is to remedy past policy mistakes that have given the elderly incentive to exit the labor force.

The last chapter—"Paying for Medicare in the Twenty-first Century," by Andrew J. Rettenmaier and Thomas R. Saving—brings together some of the issues discussed by the other authors and presents a proposal to prefund Medicare. Their work deals with all three elements of the solution space. First, by moving to a prepaid system, they fix the ratio of beneficiaries to workers at unity since each worker is paying for his or her own retirement health care. Second, by removing first-dollar coverage with the insurance they propose, both suppliers and demanders will care what health care costs, which will help control the level of benefits per person.

Their proposal is in much the same vein as proposals to prefund Social Security but with modifications to address the unique issues related to prefunding a health insurance contract. The central features of this proposal are (1) the establishment of individual retirement health insurance accounts in which contributions accumulate over individuals' years in the labor force and are used to purchase health insurance upon retirement, (2) the conversion of Medicare's two-part structure to a single higher-deductible policy for future retirees, and (3) the gradual elimination of the current federally run Medicare program.

The authors suggest that in the context of an overlapping generations model, a transition to a prefunded system from a transfer payment system will increase the capital stock. They estimate the contribution rates as a percentage of lifetime earnings, necessary to prefund two types of retirement health benefit series under a broad range of real interest rates and medical expenditure growth rates. The contribution rates for new labor force entrants are below the current implied tax rates under reasonable assumptions. The authors estimate that the transition cost associated with prefunding Medicare is substantially less than the cost of making the current pay-as-you-go system solvent. They conclude that it is thus reasonable to consider the prefunding option and present a complete transition scenario.

Chapter One

"Provide, Provide": The Economics of Aging

Victor R. Fuchs

"May you live to a hundred and twenty." This traditional Jewish blessing was inspired by the last chapter of the Torah, which describes the death of Moses at that age with "his eyes undimmed and his vigor unabated" (Deut. 34:7). Unlike Moses, many people experience a more troubled old age. In addition to the loss of family and friends and a diminution of status,[1] nearly all older persons face two potentially serious economic problems: declining earning power and increased utilization of health care. The decline in earning power is attributable to physiological changes[2] and to obsolescence of skills and knowledge, and is exacerbated by public and private policies that reduce the incentives of older persons to continue working and increase the cost to employers of employing older workers. Increased utilization of health care is undertaken to reduce or offset the effects of declining health.

The two economic problems of earnings replacement and health care payment are usually discussed separately, but there are several reasons why they should be considered together. First, there are often trade-offs between the two. Money is money, and for most people there is never enough to go around. This is self-evident where private funds are concerned. Low-income elderly, for instance, frequently must choose between expensive prescription drugs and an adequate diet.

Victor R. Fuchs is the Henry J. Kaiser Jr. Professor Emeritus at Stanford University in the Department of Economics and the Department of Health Services Research. He is also a research associate with the National Bureau of Economic Research.

I am very grateful to Deborah Kerwin-Peck for excellent research assistance. For help with the data, I thank Dan Feenberg, Eanswythe Grabowski, and Charles Nelson; the comments of Alan Krueger, Irving Leveson, Mark McClellan, James Poterba, Finis Welch, and Richard Zeckhauser are also gratefully acknowledged. Thanks are due to the Robert Wood Johnson and Andrew W. Mellon Foundations for financial support of my work.

For middle-income elderly, the choice may be between more expensive Medigap insurance and an airplane trip to a grandchild's graduation. Difficult choices are also apparent with respect to public funds. The same tax receipts that could be used to maintain or increase retirement benefits could be used to fund additional health care, and vice versa. In discussing these trade-offs, one health policy analyst asserts that people would gladly give up other goods and services for medical care that cures illness, relieves pain, or restores function (Glied 1997, 213). But the reverse is also possible. Some people may be willing to forgo some health insurance to maintain access to other goods and services.

A second reason for looking at the two problems together is that they pose similar questions for public policy: How much should each generation provide for its own needs in old age, and how much should be provided to them by their children's generation? How much provision should be voluntary, and how much compulsory? How much intragenerational redistribution is appropriate after age 65? How well can private markets serve the elderly's desire for annuities and health insurance, and when are public programs more efficient?

Finally, the magnitude of the problem of health care payment is approaching that of earnings replacement in economic importance and by 2020 will far exceed it. Declining health after age 65 results in substantial increases in the use of prescription drugs, hospital admissions, repair or replacement of parts of the body, rehabilitation and physical therapy, and assistance with daily living. New technologies offer great promise for mitigating the health problems of aging, but often at considerable expense. Overall, per capita health care expenditures after age 65 are more than three times greater than before 65 (Waldo et al. 1989).

This paper focuses primarily on the apparently relentless increase in consumption of health care by older Americans. If consumption continues to increase at the same rate as in the past, it will amount to 10 percent of the GDP by 2020, more than double the 1995 share. If the government's share of the total (about 63 percent) remains unchanged, the tax burden on younger cohorts will increase proportionately. Concomitantly, if the private share remains unchanged, income available to the elderly for other goods and services will be less in 2020 than in 1995. Although the emphasis of the chapter is on aggregate and average results for the elderly, income inequality among the elderly is also examined and compared with inequality at younger ages. The chapter concludes with a discussion of changes that might avert the economic and social crises foreshadowed by the data.

Consumption of Health Care and Income Available for Other Goods and Services

Sources and Methods

The estimates presented in table 1.1 were calculated from data obtained from a wide variety of sources. To summarize, the population data and projections (middle series) are from the Bureau of the Census. Medicare expenditures on the elderly were obtained from the Health Care Finance Administration. Total personal health care expenditures were estimated by applying ratios of total personal health care to Medicare expenditures, as presented in Waldo et al. (1989). Projected expenditures were obtained by extrapolating trends in age-specific constant-dollar expenditures and population projections.

Income available for other goods and services was estimated by subtracting personal income taxes and private health care expenditures from personal income. Taxes paid by the elderly were calculated by Dan Feenberg (1998) using the NBER tax model. Private expenditures for health care (supplementary insurance premiums plus out-of-pocket payments) were estimated using the ratios of private to total expenditures calculated by Waldo et al. Personal income was obtained from the March (of the following year) supplement of the Current Population Survey (CPS).[3] Unfortunately, there is strong evidence of underreporting of income in the CPS. The Census Bureau, using comparisons of CPS money income with independent estimates, has calculated that CPS income for the total population in 1990 was 88 percent of income calculated from independent sources. The extent of underreporting varies greatly depending on the source of the income. For example, the CPS wage and salary income is estimated to be 97 percent of the figure obtained from independent estimates, but CPS income from interest is only 51 percent of the independent estimate, and income from dividends, only 33 percent.

To show the possible effects of underreporting, two estimates of income available for other goods and services are presented, CPS and CPS-Adjusted. The adjustments were made by applying the Census

Table 1.1 Consumption of Health Care and Income Available for Other Goods and Services, Americans Ages 65 and Over

	1975	**1985**	**1995**	**2020**	**2020**
Population[a]					
Millions	22.7	28.5	33.5	53.2	53.2
As percent of total population	10.5	11.9	12.8	16.5	16.5
Medicare[b]					
Per person (dollars)	1,473	2,713	4,114	14,309[c]	11,107[d]
Total (billions)	33	77	138	762	591
As percent of GDP	0.8	1.3	1.9	5.24	4.51
Total personal health care[e]					
Per person (dollars)	3,485	6,088	9,231	29,445[c]	24,391[d]
Total (billions)	79	174	310	1,567	1,298
As percent of GDP	1.9	3.0	4.3	10.8	9.9
Income available for other goods and services[f]					
CPS					
Per person (dollars)	9,241	10,492	11,203	9,803[g]	9,059[h]
Total (billions)	210	299	376	522	482
As percent of GDP	5.0	5.2	5.2	3.6	3.7
CPS-ADJUSTED					
Per person (dollars)	13,054	16,188	15,367	14,233[g]	9,162[h]
Total (billions)	296	462	515	758	488
As percent of GDP	7.1	8.1	7.1	5.2	3.7

NOTE: All dollar amounts in 1995 dollars adjusted by the GDP implicit deflator.

[a]Population data and projections for 2020 from the U.S. Census Bureau, middle series.

[b]Health Care Financing Review Statistical Supplement 1997.

[c]Estimated from extrapolation of trend in age-specific rate of expenditures 1975–95 and Census Bureau population projections.

[d]Estimated from extrapolation of trend in age-specific rate of expenditures 1985–95 and Census bureau population projections.

[e]Estimated from relationship between total personal health care and Medicare in 1977 (for 1975) and 1987 (for 1985, 1995, and 2020) (Waldo et al. 1989).

[f]Estimated from personal income (Current Population Survey, March 1976, 1986, 1996) less taxes (Feenberg 1998) less private health care expenditures (ratios of private to total personal health care from Waldo et al. 1989).

[g]Estimated from extrapolations of 1975–95 trends in personal income and private health care expenditures.

[h]Estimated from extrapolations of 1985–95 trends in personal income and private health care expenditures.

Bureau estimates of underreporting by source of income (for all ages) to each source of income for the elderly. The adjustment factors for 1995 were the ratios of the 1990 independent estimates to the CPS incomes; for 1985, an average of the 1983 and 1987 ratios; and for 1975, the 1979 ratios (Bureau of the Census 1980, 1987, 1991, 1992). The deductions for taxes and private health care expenditures are identical for both estimates of income.

Results

The most striking result of the extrapolations is that even the more conservative one shows health care for the elderly requiring one-tenth of the GDP by 2020. Per capita consumption of health care will reach $25,000 in 1995 dollars.[4] A second important result is the dramatic effect of rising health care expenditures on income available to the elderly for other goods and services. The absolute level of residual income (in constant dollars) is projected to be lower in 2020 than in 1995; expressed as a share of GDP, the projected decrease will be even greater. This projection is based on the projections for total health care expenditures and the assumption that the ratio of private to total expenditures will be 37 percent, the same as in 1995. The projections for 2020 are not unqualified predictions. Their principal purpose is to show what will happen if the rate of health care consumption of the elderly does not slow and the rate of growth of their income does not accelerate.

Comparison of CPS and CPS-Adjusted income estimates indicates that the former may significantly understate the income of the elderly. The adjustment procedure outlined above results in an adjusted income that is 32 percent above the CPS level in 1975. The differential between adjusted and unadjusted is 38 percent in 1985 and 25 percent in 1995.[5] The adjustment process affects income available for other goods and services more than it does total income (in percentage terms) because the same amount for private health care expenditures is deducted from both the adjusted and unadjusted total incomes.

Differences by Age

Table 1.2 reproduces the key statistics of table 1.1 for three age groups (65–74, 75–84, and 85+) in 1995. Total personal health care expendi-

Table 1.2 Consumption of Health Care and Income Available for Other Goods and Services in 1995, by Age

	65–74	75–84	85+
Population (millions)	18.8	11.1	3.6
Medicare			
Per person (dollars)	3,097	4,958	6,781
Total (billions)	58	55	25
Total personal health care			
Per person (dollars)	6,183	10,572	19,358
Total (billions)	116	118	70
Income available for other goods and services			
CPS			
Per person (dollars)	13,392	9,544	5,202
Total (billions)	251	106	19
CPS-ADJUSTED			
Per person (dollars)	17,726	13,417	9,254
Total (billions)	333	150	34

SOURCES AND NOTES: See table 1.1.

tures rise sharply with age, with the oldest group consuming three times as much per person as those 65–74, and almost twice as much as those 75–84. Because persons 85 and over have such high health care expenditures (a significant portion of which must be privately financed), they have relatively little income left for other goods and services. The elderly can, of course, draw down their assets to purchase medical care and other goods and services, but the importance of this source should not be exaggerated. Only minimal financial assets are available to most of the elderly, and their willingness or ability to use their housing equity is apparently limited. Uncertainty about the length of life is a significant factor in the economic behavior of the elderly. According to one study, the annuity-like character of Social Security, Medicare, and Medicaid benefits has resulted in an increase in the propensity of older Americans to consume out of their remaining lifetime resources (Gokhale, Kotlikoff, Sabelhaus 1996).

Decomposition of Change in Personal Health Care Consumption of the Elderly

Between 1975 and 1995, personal health care consumption of the elderly rose 6.82 percent per annum in constant dollars. The average annual rate of change between 1985 and 1995 was 5.77 percent. As shown in table 1.3, these rates of change can be decomposed into three components: (1) the change in age-specific consumption per person, (2) the change in the number of elderly, and (3) the change in the age distribution of the elderly. The results of this decomposition indicate that for both time periods, the highest rate of change was in per person age-specific consumption, which was more than twice as important as the rate of change in the number of elderly. Changes in the age distribution within the 65+ population were of minor significance.[6]

The Census Bureau middle series projection of the rate of change in the number of elderly between 1995 and 2020 of 1.85 percent per annum is very close to the rate of change from 1975 to 1995. Furthermore, I estimate that rates of change of the age distribution *within* the 65+ population will have virtually zero effect on health care spending; that is, the increase in the number of old-old (85+), who are the largest consumers of health care, will be offset by a large increase in the number who are 65 to 74. By assuming the same rates of increase of age-specific health care consumption per person as prevailed in the 1975–95 and 1985–95 periods, we can project two health care consumption total

Table 1.3 Decomposition of Constant Dollar Rate of Change of Total Personal Health Care Consumption of Older Americans (Percent per Annum)

	1975–95	**1985–95**	**1995–2020**	**1995–2020**
Age-specific consumption per older person	4.65	3.89	4.65[a]	3.89[b]
Number of elderly	1.95	1.61	1.85[c]	1.85[c]
Age distribution of elderly	0.22	0.27	−0.01[d]	−0.01[d]
TOTAL CHANGE	6.82	5.77	6.49	5.73

[a]The 1975–95 trend.

[b]The 1985–95 trend.

[c]Based on U.S. Census Bureau projections.

[d]Estimated from U.S. Census Bureau age-specific projections and age-specific expenditures in 1995.

rates of change for 1995 to 2020. Extrapolation from the longer period yields a projected rate of change in health care consumption of 6.49 percent per annum; the ten-year extrapolation yields a rate of 5.73 percent per annum.

The actual level of health care spending in 2020 is subject to considerable uncertainty. The rate of growth from 1985 to 1995 was slower than in the previous decade, and it is possible that there will be additional slowing in the decades ahead. On the other hand, several special circumstances were at work during the 1985–95 period, such as the introduction of DRG (diagnosis-related group) hospital reimbursement for Medicare patients, the spread of managed care (mostly for people under age 65, but with spillover effects at all ages), the squeezing of physician incomes, and the shortening of lengths of hospital stay. It may be difficult to push these interventions much further, in which case the 1985–95 trend may understate future rates of change.

Expectations at Age 65: Life, Work, and Income

Since 1975, life expectancy at age 65 has risen appreciably, especially for men. This change in life expectancy has not been accompanied by any increase in paid work by older men, and by only a small increase for women. Thus, the number of years when income must come from sources other than employment has grown, and employment's share of total income was less in 1995 than in 1975. Tables 1.4 and 1.5 summarize these trends. The first row of table 1.4 presents life expectancy at age 65, a familiar statistic calculated from age-specific mortality rates in the year indicated. It is the mean years of life remaining for the cohort that reached age 65 (in, say, 1995) if it experienced the age-specific mortality that prevailed in 1995. Expected years of work is conceptually similar; it is obtained by combining age-specific rates of work with age-specific survival rates. It shows the years of work that the cohort that reached age 65 (in, say, 1995) would experience if the age-specific work rates and the mortality rates prevailing in 1995 continued through the lifetime of that cohort. The expected years of work are not forecasts, any more than the life expectancies are forecasts. The values could be used for forecasting purposes, however, by making assumptions about future trends in age-specific mortality and age-specific work rates.

Table 1.4 Expected at Age 65[a]

	MEN			WOMEN		
EXPECTED	**1975**	**1985**	**1995**	**1975**	**1985**	**1995**
Years of life	13.7	14.6	15.6	18.0	18.6	18.9
Years of work (FTE)[b]	2.0	1.7	1.9	0.7	0.7	1.1
Years not at work	11.7	12.9	13.7	17.3	17.9	17.8

[a]Based on survival rates and age-specific rates in the year indicated.

[b]Assuming a full-time work year of 2,000 hours.

Years of life expected at age 65 increased at a rapid pace from 1975 to 1995, more rapidly for men than for women, although the latter still enjoyed a 3.3 years' advantage over men in 1995. In contrast to life expectancy, expected years of work remained relatively constant, at about two years for men and one year for women (full-time equivalents). The number of expected years *not* at work (row 1 minus row 2) rose appreciably for men from 11.7 in 1975 to 13.7 in 1995. Women also show an increase in years *not* at work, from 17.3 to 17.8 years.

The change in life expectancy, unaccompanied by an equivalent increase in expected years of work, results in the elderly relying more on sources of income other than employment in 1995 than in 1975. Part A in table 1.5 shows the share of income derived from employment for all elderly, including those living in families with one or more members under age 65. These younger family members are more likely to be in the labor force, and this tends to increase the share of income derived from employment. Part B is limited to individuals 65 and over who do not have any family members under age 65. Both CPS and CPS-Adjusted data are shown.

Mean family income per capita is approximately the same in families with and without members under age 65, but employment's share of total income is only half as large when no family members are under age 65. The employment percent of income is lower in 1995 than in 1975 independent of the presence of family members under age 65, and this is true for both the unadjusted and adjusted data. The exceptionally low shares of employment income in 1985 are attributable to low labor force participation and to the unusually high income from interest and dividends in that year. For example, in 1985 the yield on triple-A

Table 1.5 Sources of Income of the Elderly (Ages 65+) in 1975, 1985, 1995

	PART A			PART B		
	Families with Any Elderly			Families with Only Elderly		
	1975	1985	1995	1975	1985	1995
CPS						
Mean income[a]	11,818	15,004	16,587	11,475	15,011	16,486
Percent from						
Employment[b]	26	19	21	13	9	11
Interest and dividends[c]	18	26	17	22	30	20
Pensions[d]	12	14	16	14	15	18
Social Security[e]	40	39	40	48	45	46
Other[f]	3	2	5	3	1	5
CPS-ADJUSTED						
Mean income[a]	15,630	20,700	20,751	15,743	21,369	21,008
Percent from						
Employment[b]	21	14	19	11	6	10
Interest and dividends[c]	30	38	29	35	42	32
Pensions[d]	12	15	14	13	16	15
Social Security[e]	34	31	33	39	34	37
Other[f]	3	2	5	3	1	5

NOTE: All dollar amounts in thousands of 1995 dollars adjusted by the GDP implicit deflator.
[a]Family income (from all sources) divided equally among all family members.
[b]Includes wages and salaries and nonfarm and farm self-employment income.
[c]Includes rental income.
[d]Private and public employee pensions and annuities.
[e]Social Security retirement, supplementary security, and railroad retirement.
[f]Consists primarily of various social insurance and public assistance payments.

corporate bonds was 11.4 percent compared with 7.6 percent in 1995.[7] The effect of high interest rates in 1985 is particularly strong for the CPS-Adjusted data because underreporting of interest is estimated to be considerably larger than underreporting of income from most other sources. Pension income was more important in 1995 than in 1975, while Social Security declined slightly in relative importance.

Income Inequality before and after Age 65

Contrary to what many believe,[8] income inequality among the elderly is substantially *less* than at younger ages. To measure inequality, family income is divided equally among family members to obtain individual personal income. The individuals in each of eleven age groups are then arrayed from the lowest to the highest personal income, grouped by decile, and the means of each decile calculated. The ratio of the mean of the eighth to the mean of the third decile is used to measure inequality. This comparison of the 10 percent of individuals who are in the middle of the upper half of the distribution with the 10 percent who are in the middle of the bottom half yields a robust measure of income inequality. It is relatively free of the problems of mismeasurement of income at the extremes of the distribution that can play such a large role in measures such as the Gini coefficient.

Tables 1.6, 1.7, and 1.8 show the mean income of the eighth and third deciles and their ratios for CPS and CPS-Adjusted data for 1995, 1985, and 1975. The underreporting adjustment has a greater impact at older than at younger ages because income sources such as interest and divi-

Table 1.6 Mean Income* of 8th and 3rd Deciles, by Age, 1995

	CPS			**CPS-ADJUSTED**		
AGE	**8th decile**	**3rd decile**	**8th/3rd ratio**	**8th decile**	**3rd decile**	**8th/3rd ratio**
0 to 8	13,286	3,527	3.77	14,260	3,754	3.80
9 to 16	15,126	4,674	3.24	16,375	5,062	3.23
17 to 24	18,890	5,638	3.35	20,058	5,986	3.35
25 to 32	22,876	6,815	3.36	24,374	7,277	3.35
33 to 40	22,213	7,586	2.93	23,902	8,118	2.94
41 to 48	27,030	9,909	2.73	29,665	10,686	2.78
49 to 56	31,355	10,710	2.93	34,607	11,769	2.94
57 to 64	28,108	9,285	3.03	32,396	10,428	3.11
65 to 74	20,068	8,264	2.43	24,610	9,005	2.73
75 to 84	16,988	7,697	2.21	20,442	8,427	2.43
85+	16,191	7,081	2.29	20,315	7,575	2.68
median < 65			3.13			3.17
median > = 65			2.29			2.68

*Family income divided equally among all family members.

Table 1.7 Mean Income* of 8th and 3rd Deciles, by Age, 1985

	CPS			CPS-ADJUSTED		
AGE	**8th decile**	**3rd decile**	**8th/3rd ratio**	**8th decile**	**3rd decile**	**8th/3rd ratio**
0 to 8	12,195	3,730	3.27	12,630	3,942	3.20
9 to 16	14,028	4,602	3.05	14,672	4,991	2.94
17 to 24	18,411	6,143	3.00	19,358	6,481	2.99
25 to 32	21,696	6,942	3.13	22,692	7,234	3.14
33 to 40	20,705	7,550	2.74	21,778	7,968	2.73
41 to 48	23,594	8,740	2.70	25,054	9,306	2.69
49 to 56	26,603	9,708	2.74	29,357	10,930	2.69
57 to 64	24,575	8,626	2.85	30,087	10,379	2.90
65 to 74	19,059	7,617	2.50	25,885	8,937	2.90
75 to 84	16,644	6,986	2.38	23,374	8,078	2.89
85+	16,789	6,570	2.56	23,392	7,771	3.01
median < 65			2.92			2.92
median > = 65			2.50			2.90

NOTE: All dollar amounts in thousands of 1995 dollars adjusted by the GDP implicit deflator.
*Family income divided equally among all family members.

dends (which have a high rate of underreporting) constitute a greater proportion of total income of the elderly. For the same reason, the underreporting adjustment among the elderly makes more of a difference for the eighth than for the third decile. The most important finding, however, is that in 1995 income inequality at ages 65 and over is substantially less than at younger ages in both the unadjusted and adjusted measures. Indeed, in 1995 the largest inequality among the elderly (2.43 at ages 65–74) was *less* than the smallest inequality among those under 65 (2.78 at ages 41–48).

The smaller inequality after age 65 is attributable to Social Security. If income from this source is subtracted from the mean income of the eighth and third deciles in 1995, the ratios for the remaining income soar to 6.31 (CPS) and 6.60 (CPS-Adjusted) at ages 65–74, compared with 2.43 and 2.73 when all sources are included. At older ages the leveling effect of Social Security is even greater. For those 85+ in 1995, the eighth/third decile ratios after subtracting Social Security income are 11.70 (CPS) and 12.52 (CPS-Adjusted), compared with 2.29 and 2.68 when income from all sources is considered (see table 1.9). Table 1.9

Table 1.8 Mean Income* of 8th and 3rd Deciles, by Age, 1975

	CPS			CPS-ADJUSTED		
AGE	**8th decile**	**3rd decile**	**8th/3rd ratio**	**8th decile**	**3rd decile**	**8th/3rd ratio**
0 to 8	10,525	3,866	2.72	11,093	4,219	2.63
9 to 16	11,495	4,163	2.76	12,322	4,547	2.71
17 to 24	16,227	6,203	2.62	17,369	6,731	2.58
25 to 32	17,225	6,741	2.56	18,503	7,233	2.56
33 to 40	15,036	6,050	2.49	16,035	6,511	2.46
41 to 48	18,375	7,548	2.43	19,896	8,221	2.42
49 to 56	22,172	8,771	2.53	24,302	9,893	2.46
57 to 64	20,679	7,537	2.74	24,225	9,063	2.67
65 to 74	14,811	6,273	2.36	19,540	7,522	2.60
75 to 84	12,965	5,886	2.20	17,335	7,066	2.45
85+	12,763	5,310	2.40	16,478	6,577	2.51
median < 65			2.59			2.57
median > = 65			2.36			2.51

NOTE: All dollar amounts in thousands of 1995 dollars adjusted by the GDP implicit deflator.
*Family income divided equally among all family members.

shows that Social Security's share of total income rises steadily with age, reaching about 90 percent for those in the third decile at ages 85+ and about 50 percent for those in the eighth decile. To be sure, these calculations undoubtedly overstate the extent of inequality that would exist if there were no Social Security program. Current work and savings patterns and living arrangements are influenced by the existence of Social Security; in its absence, these patterns would change. The levels of inequality now observed for individuals in their fifties and early sixties probably offer a better indication of income inequality after age 65 in a world without Social Security.

Relative inequality by age changed markedly during the period from 1975 to 1995, as can be seen in figures 1.1 and 1.2 for CPS and CPS-Adjusted data, respectively. Inequality has risen appreciably at every age below 65 but has not risen for the elderly, and at some ages has actually fallen. Similar analyses that adjust for family size by using the ratio of family income to the poverty cutoff for each family yield the same conclusion.

Table 1.9 Sources of Income of the Elderly by Age in 1995, 8th and 3rd Deciles

	65–74		75–84		85+	
CPS	**8th**	**3rd**	**8th**	**3rd**	**8th**	**3rd**
Mean income[a]	20,068	8,264	16,988	7,697	16,191	7,081
Percent from						
Employment[b]	23	11	14	5	12	4
Interest and dividends[c]	15	5	15	5	18	3
Pensions[d]	22	5	19	4	12	1
Social Security[e]	35	76	46	85	51	91
Other[f]	5	4	6	2	8	2
CPS-ADJUSTED						
Mean income[a]	24,610	9,005	20,442	8,427	20,315	7,575
Percent from						
Employment[b]	20	11	13	6	10	4
Interest and dividends[c]	26	8	25	9	30	6
Pensions[d]	20	5	17	4	10	1
Social Security[e]	30	72	40	80	42	88
Other[f]	5	4	6	2	8	2

NOTE: All dollar amounts in thousands of 1995 dollars adjusted by the GDP implicit deflator.

[a]Family income (from all sources) divided equally among all family members.

[b]Includes wages and salaries and nonfarm and farm self-employment income.

[c]Includes rental income.

[d]Private and public employee pensions and annuities.

[e]Social Security retirement, supplementary security, and railroad retirement.

[f]Consists primarily of various social insurance and public assistance payments.

Effects of Medicare on Inequality

Not only is income more equally distributed after 65 than before that age, but the Medicare program makes an additional large contribution to equality in economic well-being among the elderly. Medicare serves as a health insurance policy given to every American 65 and over. Its value each year is approximately equal to the average reimbursement per beneficiary, which amounted to $4,114 in 1995 (table 1.1). Because average reimbursement is predictably related to age, the value of the policy in 1995 could also be viewed as ranging from $3,097 for beneficiaries ages 65 to 74 to $6,781 for those ages 85 and older (table 1.2).

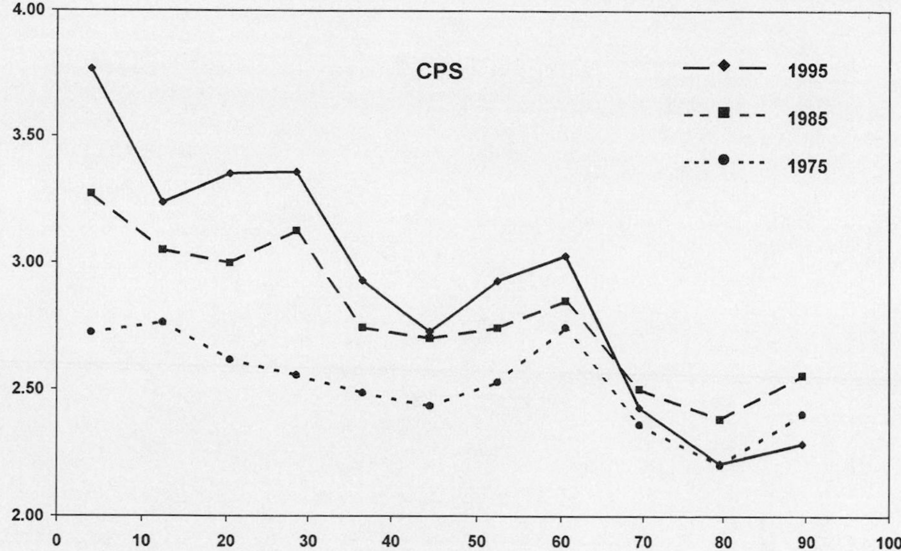

Figure 1.1 Ratio of Mean Income* of 8th to 3rd Deciles, by Age
*Family income divided equally among all family members.

Beneficiaries do pay directly for a small portion of Part B of the policy, but this is a minor offset to the value of the Medicare policy and is outweighed by the additional sales and administrative costs the elderly would have to bear if they bought a comparable policy in the private market.

If a cash transfer equal to the cost of Medicare were made to the elderly, no doubt some might choose to buy more of other goods and services instead of health insurance. Nevertheless, for the elderly as a whole, the value of the existing compulsory system may be equal to or greater than its cost because adverse selection and moral hazard would probably make a purely voluntary system unworkable. If those who did buy insurance voluntarily were above-average consumers of health care, the premium would not cover expenses and the market would tend to break down. Also, some who did not buy insurance might be relying on a socially provided "safety net" if they needed a great deal of care, thus further jeopardizing the availability of insurance for all.

When the value of Medicare is added to money income, the effect is to appreciably reduce inequality in the economic well-being of seniors.

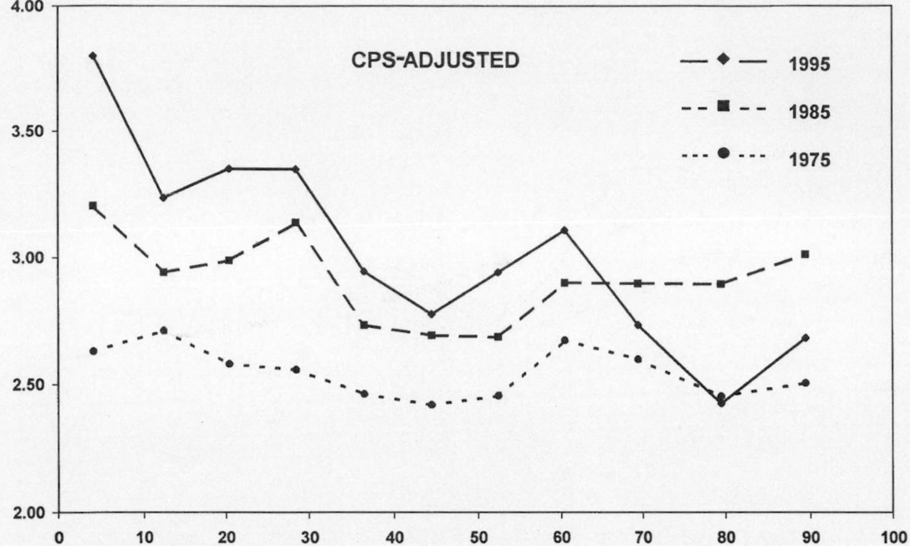

Figure 1.2 Ratio of Mean Income* of 8th to 3rd Deciles, by Age
*Family income divided equally among all family members.

The magnitude of this effect is shown in table 1.10. It is particularly large for those 85+, reflecting the greater value of Medicare relative to money income for older persons. The egalitarian thrust of Medicare reimbursements is modified slightly by the fact that average lifetime reimbursements per beneficiary tend to be larger for beneficiaries who live in higher-income areas, as identified by zip codes (McClellan and Skinner 1997).

The government also subsidizes health insurance for Americans under age 65, primarily through the tax treatment of employer contributions to premiums, but the thrust of this subsidy is much less egalitarian than that of Medicare. Many low-income workers do not benefit at all because they are not covered by private insurance. Also, workers with higher earnings tend to have more insurance than those with lower earnings. Moreover, the cash value of the tax subsidy depends on the tax bracket of the recipient—the higher the bracket, the greater the subsidy. Finally, the average value of the subsidy is small relative to the money income of persons under 65. For these reasons, the addition of the health insurance subsidy to money income for persons under 65

Table 1.10 Inequality among the Elderly in 1995, with and without the Value of Medicare

	65–74	**75–84**	**85+**
CPS			
Mean income plus Medicare*			
8th decile	23,165	21,946	22,972
3rd decile	11,361	12,655	13,862
Ratio of 8th to 3rd decile	2.04	1.73	1.66
Ratio without Medicare	2.43	2.21	2.29
CPS-ADJUSTED			
Mean income plus Medicare*			
8th decile	27,707	25,400	27,096
3rd decile	12,102	13,385	14,356
Ratio of 8th to 3rd decile	2.29	1.90	1.89
Ratio without Medicare	2.73	2.43	2.68

*Mean income from table 1.6; Medicare expenditures from table 1.2.

has a much smaller effect on economic inequality than Medicare does for persons 65 and over.

Possible Changes

The prospect of the elderly's health care consuming one-tenth of the GDP is likely to arouse considerable concern among policy makers, the public, and the elderly themselves. This is a larger share of GDP than most nations currently spend, or are planning to spend, on health care for citizens of all ages. Also, in some of these countries the elderly make up a larger percentage of the population than the 16.5 percent projected by the Census Bureau for the United States in 2020.

Although 10 percent of GDP is an enormous amount, there is no physical law or economic principle that says a nation cannot devote that amount of resources to health care for the elderly, if it chooses. No one questions the amount spent by the elderly on videotapes or computers, for example, because they are spending their own money. Similarly, if the elderly were paying for their own health care, either out of current income or with funds that they had put aside for this purpose before age 65, the public policy picture would be entirely different. Presently, however, almost two-thirds of the funds must be raised by taxes—taxes that are borne primarily by men and women under age 65. Such a large tax burden poses problems for the economy as a whole and could also contribute to intergenerational tension and hostility. Moreover, if the government's share of the elderly's health care bill remains the same (or decreases), the huge absolute rise in private expenditures will leave the elderly with an ever-decreasing ability to purchase other goods and services.

What economic changes could alter these results? The answers lie in three directions: (1) a decrease in the rate of growth of age-specific health care expenditures, (2) an increase in the amount of paid work by persons 65 and older, and/or (3) an increase in the savings rate of persons under age 65.

Age-specific Expenditures

The increase in health care expenditures for persons 65 and over is *not* primarily a demographic phenomenon (table 1.3). There has been and will continue to be some growth in the number of elderly, but more than two-thirds of expenditure growth has come from an increase in age-specific expenditures. Why did older persons use so much more health care in 1995 than in 1975 or 1985? Certainly not because they were sicker in 1995. On the contrary, most experts believe that the elderly are healthier now than at any previous time. The most objective evidence of this comes from mortality rates. Age-specific mortality of the elderly was appreciably higher in 1975 than in 1995—and most people are sick before they die.[9]

There is substantial consensus among health care experts that the driving force behind increasing health expenditures is new technology—new methods of diagnosis, new drugs, new surgical procedures, and the like. In a survey of fifty leading health economists in 1995, more than four out of five agreed with the statement "The primary reason for the increase in the health sector's share of GDP over the past 30 years is technological change in medicine" (Fuchs 1996).

Can the pace of technological change in medicine be slowed? Public policy can affect the development and diffusion of new medical technologies in three ways. First, the government has a huge effect on the demand for medical care through Medicare, Medicaid, and other public programs. What the government pays for and how much it pays directly influence the adoption of new technologies by health care providers and indirectly influence the amount and direction of private R&D. Second, the government heavily subsidizes the training of specialists and subspecialists, who then become important agents in the process of technology development and diffusion. Finally, the government influences technology through direct subsidization of medical research. In my judgment this is probably the least important influence, as evidenced by the lower levels of technology utilization in Canada and Western Europe compared with the United States. The results of U.S. government–subsidized research are known in all these countries, but the lower percentage of physicians who are specialists and the limitations in government funding of health care facilities and programs result in less use of expensive technology and in a lower rate of health care spending.

The example of other countries shows that public policy can slow the pace of technological change and diffusion. But does the United States want to do that? Technological innovations have contributed to longer and especially better quality of life for many older Americans. Some current research suggests that new medical technology has been cost-effective—its benefits exceed its costs. Some technological innovations lower the cost of treating a patient with a particular disease. It is a grave mistake, however, to think that lowering the cost per unit will lead to lower overall expenditures. The experience in medical care to date (and in many other industries such as personal computers) is that total expenditures increase even as cost per unit goes down. If the growth of medical expenditures continues, however, who will pay for the increase? What new sources of funds could become available to help the elderly finance medical care and also maintain their access to other goods and services?

More Work and More Saving

One possibility is greater participation in paid work by older men and women. As seen in table 1.4, employment after age 65 was about the same in 1995 as in 1975 despite substantial improvement in the health of the elderly and longer life expectancy.[10] According to one authority on retirement, better health has not prevented a long-term trend toward early retirement (Costa 1998, 195). Another recent study, however, states that this trend ended abruptly in 1985 (Quinn et al. forthcoming). Table 1.4 does show a small increase in years of work expected at age 65 between 1985 and 1995. Although the health of the elderly is improving, there are two major impediments to working after age 65. First, older workers are discouraged by the high marginal tax rates implicit in means-tested benefit structures. Second, employers often find older workers add disproportionately to their health insurance and pension costs. To increase labor force participation after age 65, policy makers will need to address both of these obstacles.

Because their own employment income accounts for a relatively small part of the total income of the elderly (10 percent in 1995), there would have to be a substantial increase in labor force participation to make a significant impact on the ability of the elderly to pay for more medical care and maintain access to other goods and services. Another possibility is for those who will reach 65 in 2020 or beyond to begin now to substantially increase their rate of saving. Income from savings (interest, dividends, and pensions) is more than four times as important as employment as a source of income after age 65. Thus, a substantial increase in this source would have a major effect on the financial condition of the elderly.

One probable side effect of an increase in the relative importance of income from employment and savings would be somewhat more income inequality among the elderly. The more voluntary the additional savings and the more individual discretion over the way the savings are invested, the greater will be the increase in inequality. But voluntary or compulsory, individually controlled or not, the clearest implication of the projections for 2020 is the need for additional savings.

This was the advice given by Robert Frost in 1936 in his poem "Provide, Provide," a portion of which follows:

> . . .
> Die early and avoid the fate.
> Or, if predestined to die late,
> Make up your mind to die in state.
> . . .
> No memory of having starred
> Atones for later disregard
> Or keeps the end from being hard.

Better to go down dignified
With boughten friendship at your side
Than none at all. Provide, provide!*

Notes

1. My wife tells participants in her preretirement workshops that it is often painful to go from *Who's Who* to "Who's he?"

2. For example, loss of strength, dexterity, stamina, sensory perceptions, cognitive functions.

3. All summary measures of income were obtained from individual records, appropriately weighted to take account of oversampling in the CPS. The data were extracted using CPS Utilities (1997).

4. All dollar figures in this paper are in 1995 dollars, using the GDP implicit price deflator as the source of adjustment.

5. If underreporting by source of income is different for the elderly than for the population as a whole, these adjustments may be too large or too small. Also, there is no certainty that the independent estimates are correct. Therefore, both CPS and CPS-Adjusted are shown throughout the paper.

6. Interactions among these terms were minuscule.

7. These are nominal yields that reflect the impact of inflation on interest rates.

8. Richard Disney (1996) states, "The income distribution of the elderly (65+) is more unequal than that of those under 65" (11). The author relies on Michael Hurd's review article (1990), which summarizes the results of earlier studies based on data for 1967, 1979, and 1984.

9. Paradoxically, good health can often lead to greater health care utilization by the elderly. Those in good health may be deemed better candidates for expensive surgical procedures that would be regarded as medically inappropriate for persons of similar age who are in poor health.

10. At any given point in time, persons in poorer health tend to retire earlier (Dwyer and Mitchell 1998).

References

Bureau of the Census. *Money Income of Households, Families, and Persons in the United States: 1980, 1987, 1991, and 1992.* Tables A2 and C1.

Costa, Dora L. 1998. *The Evolution of Retirement: An American Economic History, 1880–1990.* Chicago: University of Chicago Press.

CPS Utilities. 1997. March CPS Utilities, 1964–1996, Release 96.1. Unicon Research Corporation, 1640 Fifth Street, Santa Monica, CA 90401; 310-393-4636.

Disney, Richard. 1996. *Can We Afford to Grow Older? A Perspective on the Economics of Aging.* Cambridge: MIT University Press.

Dwyer, Debra Sabatini, and Olivia Mitchell. 1998. "Health Problems as Determinants of Retirement: Are Self-Rated Measures Endogenous?" NBER Working Paper 6503 (April).

Feenberg, Dan. 1998. Personal communication.

Frost, Robert. "Provide, Provide." In *The Norton Anthology of Modern Poetry*, 2d ed., edited by Richard Ellman and Robert O'Clair. New York: W. W. Norton, 1988, p. 263.

Fuchs, Victor R. 1996. "Economics, Values, and Health Care Reform." *American Economic Review* 86 (1, March): 1–24.

Glied, Sherry. 1997. *Chronic Condition: Why Health Reform Fails.* Cambridge: Harvard University Press.

Gokhale, Jagadeesh, Laurence Kotlikoff, and John Sabelhaus. 1996. "Understanding the Postwar Decline in U.S. Saving: A Cohort Analysis." *Brookings Papers on Economic Activity* (1).

Hurd, Michael. 1990. "Research on the Elderly: Economic Status, Retirement, and Consumption and Saving." *Journal of Economic Literature* 28 (2, June).

McClellan, Mark, and Jonathan Skinner. 1997. "The Incidence of Medicare." NBER mimeo (April), p. 21.

Quinn, Joseph F., Richard Burkhauser, Kevin Cahill, and Robert Weathers. Forthcoming. "The Microeconomics of the Retirement Decision in the United States." OECD Working Paper, Paris.

Waldo, Daniel R., Sally T. Sonnefeld, David R. McKusick, and Ross H. Arnett III. 1989. "Health Expenditures by Age Group, 1977 and 1987." *Health Care Financing Review* 10 (4, summer): 116–20 (see table 4, p. 118).

Chapter Two

Medicare Choice: Good, Bad, or It All Depends

Henry J. Aaron

Any expansion of personal choice under the new system is a good thing.
—Robert Moffitt, Heritage Foundation

There may be a lot of confusion.
—Bruce Vladeck, former commissioner of the Health Care Financing Administration

Managed care scares the hell out of me.
—Eileen Logan, sixty-six-year-old retired Boeing engineer

Freedom of choice is a good thing—potentially.
—Judith Feder, Georgetown University[1]

For those involved in the financing and delivery of health care services, the old saw "God save me from living in interesting times" could hardly be more apt. Revolutionary advance of medical technology is not new, but neither is it slowing. The reorganization of the delivery of health care is so rapid that today's organization charts molder in months. Physicians form new groups. Hospitals merge and close. Health insurers, hospital chains, and managed care organizations catapult into the Fortune 1000, whereupon some stumble, some get swallowed up, and others just keep on enrolling patients. Insured individuals find themselves subject to new rules and restrictions. The relationships of the insured to their insurers and of health care providers to their payers have

Henry J. Aaron is the Bruce and Virginia MacLaury Senior Fellow, Economic Studies Program, the Brookings Institution.

I wish to thank Robert Reischauer and Charles Schultze for helpful criticisms on an earlier draft.

changed more in the past five years than they did cumulatively since health insurance became commonplace in the 1950s.

A leading characteristic of developments in health care is the increasing exercise of choice (1) by companies in selecting health plans in which employees may enroll; (2) by plan managers in picking providers and setting guidelines for care, including limitations on patients' access to providers, diagnostic procedures, and therapies; and (3) by individuals in selecting health plans from the menu of plans designated by their employers. The principle underlying this system is that choice, as exercised in the first instance by employers and ultimately by covered individuals, will drive competition among risk bearers and care providers (sometimes, but not always, the same entity), which are free to enter and to exit from particular activities and to choose how to organize themselves and what services to provide. To be sure, choice exercised at one level in the system may narrow choice at another. Such downstream narrowing of choice occurs when companies curtail options of their employees to stay with a particular physician by switching from an unrestricted fee-for-service plan to a managed preferred provider plan or to an HMO. It also occurs when the insured voluntarily limit future options by joining plans that limit access to providers by establishing gatekeepers or using strict case management. HMO rules on mental health services clearly illustrate such limits. To a considerable extent, employers are making decisions on behalf of employees that limit choice on the ground that the benefits from reducing (the growth) of spending will outweigh any limits on care—and may improve care in some cases. On balance, the emergence of managed care has probably reduced the range of choice in health care by individuals. Nonetheless, the rationale behind the transformation of the financing and delivery of health care is the belief that individuals, if forced to bear the financial consequences of choosing higher-cost health plans, will make choices that promote competition among risk bearers and health care providers, and that increased competition will ultimately bring about an improved balance of social costs and social benefits from health care. This division of responsibility raises obvious principle/agent problems.

A health care program as large as Medicare could not possibly escape these developments. Since 1982 Medicare enrollees have had the option to join health maintenance organizations in communities where HMOs exist and have elected to participate in the Medicare program.[2] The Balanced Budget Act of 1997 initiated a new era of expanded options for Medicare beneficiaries. Under this law, health care insurers and providers are encouraged to provide services under several different arrangements that will dramatically expand the scope of choice regarding health plan management for Medicare eligibles.

The new legislation raises important structural questions:

- Will reforms enacted in 1997, which expand choice under Medicare, facilitate the further modifications in the program that most observers believe will be necessary as health care arrangements for the rest of the population change, as the flood of baby boomers becomes eligible for Medicare and pushes up costs, and as medical technology continues to evolve?
- Will the expansion of choice benefit participants? This question can be taken in several senses. Will the new arrangements lower Medicare costs? Will they lower the costs of providing care of a given quality? Will they increase patient satisfaction? Will they raise or lower clinical quality?
- Is the extension of choice in Medicare, and in health care generally, a good thing?

I will take up these questions in reverse order.

- On the question of whether extension of choice is a good thing in general, the answer is (as it always must be): It all depends. In some quarters, a view seems to have taken hold that anything that promotes choice or competition is necessarily benign. This view is bad economic *theory* for reasons I present below. Whether adding choice and promoting competition are good *policy* always depends on what lawyers call "facts and circumstances," which include the nature and structure of markets and the way competition is structured.
- On the second question, the jury is still out. Evidence is fairly clear that, as implemented so far, choice has raised Medicare costs in a way I will explain presently. We still do not know whether the extension of choice in Medicare, when proper financing mechanisms are in place, will lower or raise overall costs of providing health care to the Medicare population or promote efficient provision of services. We also do not have better than provisional answers on how choice will affect patient satisfaction and clinical quality of care. Actually, the jury has not yet been impaneled as this paper is written, because the results depend on how regulations to implement the Balanced Budget Act of 1997 are written and how an extremely dynamic market responds.

- On the first question, the 1997 Medicare reforms are likely to hinder rather than facilitate further reforms in Medicare. This conclusion is somewhat paradoxical. For reasons I will explain below, I believe that it will be necessary to liberalize and standardize Medicare benefits in order to give competitive markets a chance to function well. The 1997 reforms are likely to raise the budget cost of implementing such a benefit package and, therefore, make it politically more difficult to enact.

Before addressing these three questions in detail, however, I briefly outline the current options in Medicare coverage and the new options contained in the 1997 legislation.

Choice in Medicare

In 1982 Congress authorized Medicare beneficiaries to enroll in managed care organizations operating under so-called "risk contracts." Under these contracts, providers accept capitation and provide *at least* the range of services promised under traditional Medicare. Risk contracts may cover standard closed-panel services of health maintenance organizations or point-of-service plans. Since 1982 Medicare has paid risk contractors 95 percent of average local costs of caring for participants under the basic program.

Most Medicare risk plans provide more services than Medicare requires (see table 2.1). Risk contractors can afford to provide extra ser-

Table 2.1 Additional Services Offered by Medicare Risk HMOs

Service	**Percent of HMOs offering (November 1997)**
Routine physicals	97
Eye examinations	92
Ear examinations	78
Immunizations	89
Outpatient drugs	68
Health education	37
Dental services	39
Foot care	30

SOURCE: American Association of Health Plans

vices for 5 percent less than the average cost of Medicare for several reasons. First, some managed care providers can provide mandated services at lower cost than can fee-for-service providers. Second, the capitation rate is much higher in some regions than in others, relative to properly measured local costs of care. In 1997 the average adjusted monthly cost of Medicare ranged from $221 to $767 (National Academy of Social Insurance 1998). Substantial differences occur even between neighboring counties in metropolitan areas. Quite naturally, risk contracts are most frequent in areas with relatively high payment levels. In 1994, estimated payment per beneficiary enrolled in risk contracts was $3,963, compared with an estimated outlay of $3,656 if these people had remained in traditional Medicare.[3] Third, risk contractors have proven adept at enrolling members with lower-than-average medical costs and in driving away members with higher-than-average costs. The Medicare Payment Advisory Commission reports that in the six months before enrolling in managed care plans, beneficiaries' costs were 37 percent below those for a fee-for-service comparison group. In the six months after disenrolling, beneficiaries' costs were 60 percent above the fee-for-service average (LeRoy, Hoadley, and Merrell 1997).

Because of the highly skewed nature of the distribution of payments, potential profits in risk selection are vast. Nearly 20 percent of Medicare enrollees generate no costs in a given year while the upper 10 percent of beneficiaries generate 75 percent of the costs (see figure 2.1) (Komisar et al. 1997). The Medicare program deals with this skewness by basing Medicare payments to risk contractors on the age, sex, Medicaid status, institutional status, and employment status of enrollees, which erodes potential profits from selecting patients from low-cost categories. But these adjusters account for less than 5 percent of the variance in annual outlays. Large potential profits remain because plans can use marketing devices to appeal to potential enrollees with low expected costs and because health plans acquire proprietary information about enrollees.[4] However, the fact that most variance is random and unpredictable given current information does place strict limits on the potential of risk selection.

The proportion of Medicare patients served under risk contracts has been small, but growth accelerated in the mid-1990s. As of November 1997, 307 plans served 5.7 million people—less than one Medicare enrollee in seven but 25 percent more than one year earlier. Enrollment in risk contracts was geographically concentrated—the proportion en-

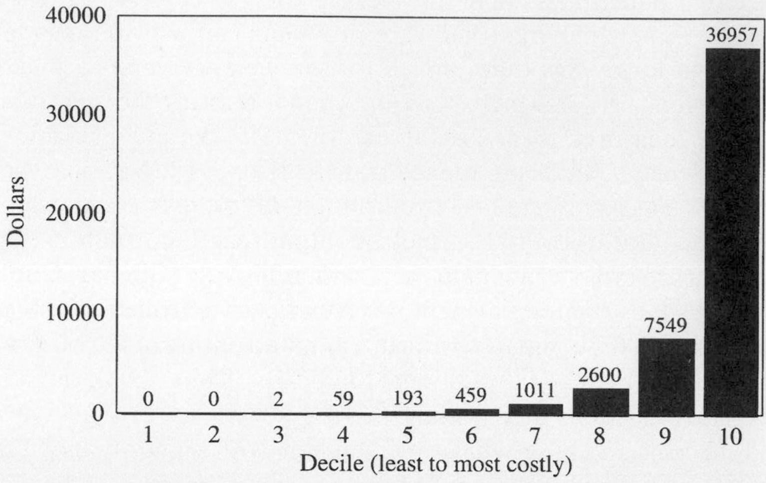

Figure 2.1 Medical Expenditures per Beneficiary by Decile, 1996
SOURCE: Marilyn Moon, "Restructuring Medicare's Cost Sharing," *The Commonwealth Fund* (December 1996).

rolled in risk contracts is 20 percent or more of Medicare eligibles in seven states but 5 percent or less in twenty-seven states. Half of all enrollees in plans with risk contracts lived in California, Florida, and Pennsylvania (American Association of Health Plans 1998).

Criticisms of the system used to pay risk contractors abound. Payments vary enormously not only from area to area, but also from year to year. The temporal variation arises primarily in small counties. Average fee-for-service Medicare costs are driven everywhere by a small proportion of particularly costly cases. In small counties, a given absolute deviation is relatively more important than in large markets. Geographical variability explains why enrollment in risk contracts is high in some places and nonexistent in others. In high-payment areas, risk contractors can provide, in addition to the basic Medicare benefit package, extra services for which enrollees in traditional Medicare have to pay out-of-pocket or buy supplemental (Medigap) coverage. Where payments are low, HMOs cannot afford to offer even the basic benefit package and none has entered the market.

A second criticism of the current system arises from the fact that risk adjustments in payments to risk contractors offset only about 5 percent of the variance in actual Medicare expenditures. As a result, risk contractors have had large incentives to enroll low-cost enrollees and to drive relatively high-cost members back to the traditional Medicare program. Moreover, as I have noted, they have proven adept at doing exactly that.

The Balanced Budget Act of 1997 legislation created several additional alternatives to traditional Medicare, collectively named Medicare+Choice. Up to 390,000 Medicare participants will be able to combine high-deductible insurance (up to $6,000 a year) with tax-sheltered savings accounts—medical savings accounts (MSAs). The MSA balances may be used to pay for medical expenses or, if the balance exceeds 60 percent of the deductible, for other purposes. If the balance is less than 60 percent of the deductible, a penalty tax will apply to withdrawals for nonmedical purposes. In addition to MSAs, the 1997 legislation authorizes groups of physicians, or other providers, to set up provider-sponsored organizations (PSOs) to cover Medicare eligibles. It also authorizes the creation of private fee-for-service plans that may offer any of a wide range of benefit packages at least as generous as Medicare, possibly limited to very generous plans that require substantial payment by enrollees in addition to the Medicare subvention.[5]

Medicare will make capitation payments on behalf of Medicare eligibles to organizations that run these new options. The payments will at first be based on local costs of care (but the weighting of local costs will diminish) and some personal characteristics of those who enroll in MSAs, HMOs, and PSOs. Largely because of adverse selection, the Congressional Budget Office estimates that MSAs and PSOs will *increase* total Medicare spending. MSA plans are also expected to attract relatively healthy enrollees, although the absence of protection regarding physician fees may limit MSA appeal. Physicians who set up PSOs are expected to send their relatively healthy patients to these organizations and encourage sicker patients to remain under traditional Medicare. The record of risk contractors to date supports these assumptions. If Medicare were able to predict medical outlays accurately for individuals or institute risk adjustments that control for a higher proportion of the variance in Medicare expenditures, it could take enough of the profit out of risk selection to make this form of competition unappealing. Because the Health Care Financing Administration currently lacks such capacity, the Congressional Budget Office expects Medicare payments to MSAs and PSOs to exceed the cost of care that enrollees in these plans would otherwise have used.

The expected inflationary effect of choice on Medicare costs is "inflation-in-the-small," which means that costs will be higher than they would be under traditional Medicare, *all other aspects of the system of health care financing and delivery held constant*. However, as I have indicated, nothing these days is constant in health care finance and delivery. The introduction of increased choice and of managed care throughout the health care system has probably contributed to the reduction in growth of overall spending by pressuring providers to close excess capacity, operate more efficiently, squeeze out rents, and hold down prices. If one accepts the view that choice and the competitive environment it fosters has helped produce "deflation-in-the-large," the introduction of choice in Medicare is part of that change in the environment determining health care spending. In that event, Medicare costs might be higher or lower if only traditional fee-for-service Medicare were available. I know of no research that enables one to distinguish deflation-in-the-large from inflation-in-the-small or to measure their relative size.

To reduce huge geographic and temporal variation in payments, Congress in 1997 established a floor on payments under risk contracts and Medicare+Choice. It also decreed that payments on behalf of enrollees who leave traditional Medicare are to be based on both local costs and national average cost, equally weighted. As a result, payments on behalf of patients who leave traditional Medicare will rise sharply—by as much as 40 to 50 percent in some counties. HMOs, PPOs, PSOs, and private fee-for-service plans are likely to spring up in many areas where capitated plans did not find operations feasible in the past. In fact, payments in some places will considerably exceed those made under traditional Medicare. This situation creates the possibility of a paradoxical asymmetry—more inflation-in-the-small and deflation-in-the-large.

Medicare enrollees appeared to sacrifice their freedom to choose providers and accepted limits on care by enrolling in HMOs and other plans with closed panels and tight case management. In fact, enrollees have not in the past actually given up very much. Before the new rules contained in the Balanced Budget Act of 1997 take effect, enrollees could disenroll from an HMO and rejoin traditional Medicare on a monthly basis. All HMOs had to offer at least a month-long open enrollment period annually, and many accepted enrollees at any time. The Balanced Budget Act of 1997 sets gradually tighter *legal* limits on the frequency with which HMO enrollees will be allowed to return to traditional Medicare. By 2003 patients will effectively be bound to a plan for nearly one year, but annual choice will remain an option, as under most private plans.[6]

Market developments may well close off some options. For example, the options that the 1997 legislation creates for physicians to set up new modes of serving Medicare patients may cause traditional fee-for-service medicine in thinly settled areas to become unavailable. This outcome would follow if most physicians in a particular geographical area elect to see patients only under new insurance arrangements that enable them to make higher incomes than current arrangements make possible. If managed care plans were able to predict in advance the exact medical costs of every enrollee and were able to enroll only the least costly, *n* percent of patients, the average cost of fee-for-service Medicare would explode as *n* increases (see figure 2.2). This degree of risk selection is infeasible, but a cost spiral based on more limited risk selection is not, especially in small areas.

In summary, providing Medicare enrollees the option of shifting

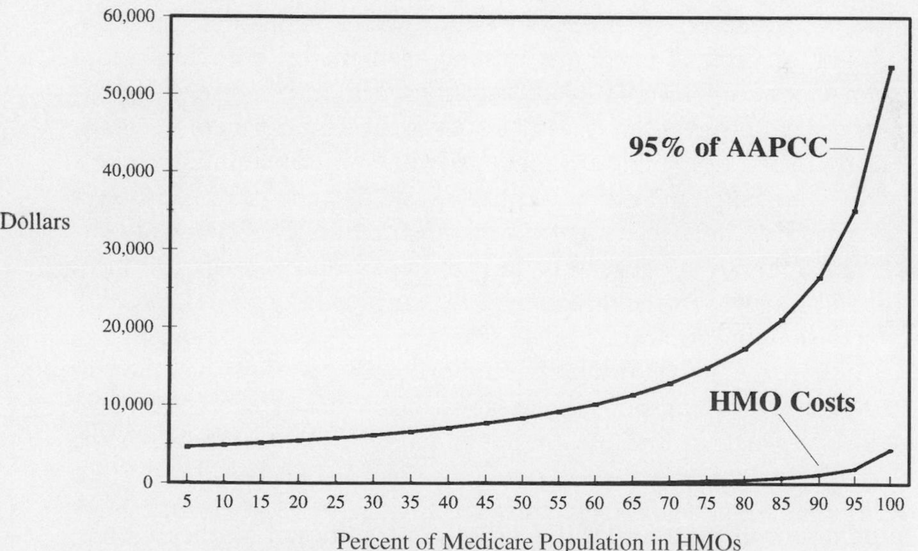

Figure 2.2 HMO Revenues and Costs per Beneficiary as HMO Participation Rate Increases—"Perfect" Risk Selection

Prepared by Robert Reischauer

from traditional fee-for-service Medicare has raised and will raise program costs (but may, perhaps, have contributed to institutional changes that many credit with slowing growth of total health care spending). The effect of these options on total health care spending on behalf of Medicare enrollees is less clear. Some of the added program costs caused by risk contracting and anticipated for Medicare+Choice have enabled risk contractors to provide services for which individuals would otherwise have paid directly or bought indirectly through Medigap coverage. The result could easily be a drop in out-of-pocket costs for enrollees and lower total system costs. In addition, HMO risk contractors may produce health services more cheaply than fee-for-service providers do. Little is known about the overall effect of risk contracts on the quality of care or (cost-adjusted) patient satisfaction.

Competition and Choice

As the twentieth century wanes, governments and intellectuals around the world are recoiling from a nearly century-long experiment with government ownership of major industries and central economic planning. The collapse of the Soviet Union and its epigones; the catastrophic records of economic mismanagement by governments in Latin America, Africa, and, most recently, Asia; and the general inefficiency of state-run enterprises all testify to the superiority of free markets for promoting stable economic growth. Well-functioning markets require free entry and exit by companies and free choice by consumers and producers, all backed up by good information. The spread of market principles in the last years of the twentieth century is one of the most hopeful auguries for improvement in worldwide economic welfare over the coming decades.

At the same time, however, it is important that the lesson of the failures of governmental obtrusiveness and the virtues of markets not lead to an overreaction. Specifically, not all measures that promote choice and competition necessarily promote welfare. In fact, we all know that well-functioning markets actually require intrusive government actions—to establish a strict and just rule of law, to establish property rights, to help establish institutions that minimize transaction costs, to regulate economic activities where unfettered markets have led to abuses, to avoid the various tragedies of the commons, and to cushion the effects of the competitive struggle on the unlucky or unskilled. Restricting government interference in the economy that effectively addresses these shortcomings would lower welfare and market efficiency, not promote them.

Nonetheless, some participants in the health policy debate seem to embrace the view that any action that adds to choice is desirable. Behind this belief seems to lie a tacit syllogism:

Policy A will increase choice.
Increasing choice promotes competition.
Competition raises welfare.
Therefore: Policy A will raise welfare (at least if the market sustains it).

This line of reasoning seems simple and straightforward. At the consumer level, providing people a new choice gives them access to something that was not previously available. If consumers reject the option, no harm, it seems, is done. If they elect it, they reveal themselves to be better off. No one loses and some may gain. Adding choices that *anyone* selects, it would seem, must increase consumer welfare. On the supply side, the reasoning is similar. Adding choice reduces the capacity of suppliers to extort rents from buyers and thereby helps lower the level, if not the rate of growth, of production costs and align market prices with social cost. Choice encourages economy in the provision of services. Those who use this argument seem to regard it as too obvious to require explicit argument.

These simple principles contain much wisdom. Every economics student learns them in the first few weeks of any principles course worth the time it takes to enroll. Applied to health care, these principles help observers understand why people value choice among alternative insurance packages and unfettered access to a large roster of physicians. They also help explain why barriers to entry into medicine prop up the prices that practitioners can charge and why the expiration of drug patents typically leads to lower prices.

Slightly more advanced economic theory reveals that restricting choice may occasionally improve welfare. Granting of patents, for example, encourages innovation, which may be worth more than the costs of monopoly pricing. Increased choice can also reduce consumer welfare and may raise costs. The complexity of health insurance contracts, for example, creates a hard choice between the unfettered freedom of risk bearers to tailor insurance packages to the desires of particular customers and the capacity of customers to choose among dozens of plans with differences both gross and subtle. In extreme cases, increasing choice can cause previously well-functioning markets to fail.

Insights from psychology and behavioral economics provide additional reasons why, in plausible situations, increased choice can create more problems than it solves. What all this means is that the conclusion "Increased choice is good for welfare" is not a logical truth, but an empirical proposition. Observing that some policy promotes choice is not sufficient proof that the policy is benign. In much the same sense, however, observing that some market is functioning in a less-than-perfect way is not sufficient proof that interfering with the market will raise welfare.

I turn now to several classes of reasons that should cause health care policy makers to look carefully at facts and circumstances in deciding whether increased choice is desirable and to pay careful attention to market rules and regulations. As will become apparent, these categories overlap and blur into one another. I want to emphasize at the outset that some of these considerations rest on unabashed paternalism. Regulations or rules may spare people from making decisions—such as going without health insurance—that they will later regret or find costly or impossible to reverse. Nor is regret about past error necessary for the conclusion that choice lowers welfare. A social judgment may be reached that well-informed individual decisions that the decider never regrets are not legitimate and should be prevented. For example, there is a continuing tension between the unfettered rights of individuals to make decisions for "dependents"—children or incompetent adults—and the supervisory role of society in assuring that dependents are not abused.

I want to make clear that the examples that follow establish only that increased choice in particular aspects of the market for health care services *may* produce inferior results for identifiable reasons. Limits on choice should only be adopted when they are shown to produce superior results. And, given the records of market and nonmarket decision making in recent decades, the burden of proof should rest with those who would abridge market processes.

Fallible Reasoning, Changing Preferences

Economists have customarily assumed that individuals efficiently process available information to maximize stable preferences. A mountain of research by psychologists, sociologists, experimental economists, information theorists, and logicians has established that this assumption is descriptively false—not just a bit off the mark, but massively inaccurate. In fact, rational reasoning in the sense of applying the laws of logic to available information is physically impossible for humans to achieve. In the case of health care, Oaksford and Chater (1993) observe:

> Diagnoses involving just two symptoms, together with some reasonable assumptions concerning the numbers of diseases and symptoms a physician may know about, require upwards of 109 numbers to be stored in memory. Since typical diagnoses may work on upwards of 30 symptoms, even if every connection in the human brain were encoding a digit, its capacity would nonetheless be exceeded. Such complexity considerations render it highly unlikely that human decision makers are generally employing Bayesian decision theory in their risky decision making. Such results were primarily responsible for the emergence of the heuristics-and-biases approach in the psychology of human decision making. (37)

Problems that individuals routinely encounter are computationally insoluble in reasonable lengths of time with the mental machinery humans possess. Problems can be classified on the basis of their complexity, defined by the number of steps in solutions in "worst case" situations. In certain problems, the minimum number of steps necessary to assure a solution can become so large that sufficient time does not exist for even the most rapid computer, operating since the beginning of the universe, to have solved the problem.[7]

Because people constantly deal with problems they cannot solve analytically, they use rules of thumb and shortcuts that on the average work well in circumstances in which the rules evolved. Unfortunately, these rules, which become habitual and hard to dislodge, may fail systematically and grossly in new circumstances. For example, the brain employs various rules of thumb to construct mental images from the cacophony of optical stimuli. These rules of thumb have evolved over eons and clearly have survival value in most natural circumstances. When these circumstances change—as they can be made to change in the researcher's laboratory—the result is an optical illusion. Similar errors occur when problems arise naturally that are unlike the behavioral rules of inference people customarily employ. Furthermore, psychological research has shown that decisions do not emerge consistently based on objective circumstances. Rather, they may vary enormously depending on procedures used for eliciting the decision: whether the decision is framed as a loss or as a gain; what the decision maker's transitory visceral states happen to be at the time decisions are made; and what may seem to be tiny, seemingly irrelevant situational factors.[8] Training can reduce such biases. However, experts seem as prone to framing errors as novices.

More to the point, decisions of great importance are often ones that people make infrequently and for which training is therefore either impractical or simply not given. The menu of choices that individuals now face in selecting insurance plans is bewildering and easily rises to the complexity that Oaksford and Chater describe. Furthermore, even in simple cases, the addition of choice seems to cause people to violate the laws of rational choice. Several experiments have shown that if people are given the choice between two objects, A and B, the proportion of people favoring A *increases* if a new choice, C, is added that is identical to neither A nor B, but more closely resembles B than A.

Economic analysis, especially empirical research, traditionally has also paid little attention to the direct influence on individual preferences of the behavior and opinions of others.[9] Despite inaccurate assumptions and inattention to social interaction, the standard assumptions of economic analysis have proven useful in theoretical and empirical work. A debate has emerged on whether economic analysis would now gain added power from incorporating the research findings of psychology and sociology, at least for certain classes of problems (Akerlof 1984; Becker 1996; Simon 1986; Aaron 1994). Since all research advances on the back of simplifying assumptions, the practical question for research is not whether simplification is useful—it almost always is not only useful, but *essential*—but whether modifying the assumptions used in economic analysis to recognize research findings from psychology and sociology can improve the research. As always, the burden of proof rests, as it should, on those who propose to disturb established practices.

Whatever the results of this debate, however, a quite different question faces those who develop public policy, in general, and Medicare policy, in particular: Will individuals who are given the power to exercise choice exercise it in a way that promotes welfare, on the average? What limits on choice, if any, have the potential to increase welfare? It is worth noting that legal doctrine is not consistent in enforcing expressed preferences. Contracts on some matters can be irrevocable—donations of property, for example—but others cannot—living wills and durable powers of attorney, for example. As the Balanced Budget Act of 1997 makes clear, this issue is very much alive regarding the matter of health insurance. The act limits the freedom of enrollees in managed care plans to withdraw from them. The justification is that such limits will increase the likelihood that competition will improve welfare. Whether such freedom to choose should be unfettered, limited, or abrogated is clearly a matter of facts and circumstances, not logic or first principles.

Nonexistence of Equilibrium

Two decades have passed since Joseph Stiglitz and Michael Rothschild (1976) showed that individual freedom to decide whether to buy insurance and which plan to select might cause markets to cycle chaotically or fail altogether. No equilibrium might exist in markets for insurance even though everyone would like to buy insurance at prices that would generate profits for insurers, because insurers cannot effectively price discriminate. The problem arises because insurers have imperfect information about the expected costs and preferences of potential customers. In particular, average cost pricing within risk classes means that customers within a given risk class who have low expected costs may elect disproportionately to drop insurance coverage. Their decision boosts costs for the remaining members of that class. As the premium increases, some additional customers may drop coverage, and so on until the market implodes.

It is also possible for a single insurance plan to be economically viable, but only if customers have no choice of alternative plans. When insurers can create new plans, they can tailor them to attract lower-than-average-cost customers, driving up costs under the original plan. As customers shift to the new plan, however, it too becomes vulnerable to this strategy. In such cases, welfare may be higher if insurance options are limited to a single plan, possibly with mandatory participation, than from free choice among alternative plans.

Even if choice does not cause market failure, selective enrollment and disenrollment can produce the sort of problematic cost shifting that has resulted under Medicare risk contracts. Improved capacity to predict expected medical costs could ameliorate or eliminate the *ex ante* version of this problem by enabling insurers to charge each customer a premium equal to expected medical costs. Such premium variation would require that insurers have information about expected medical costs that is at least as good as the information people use in selecting among plans *and* that they act on this information in setting premiums. Even if insurers had such information, which none now has, they might not be able to act on it. Excessive implementation costs or political resistance to implied premium variations could force insurers to ignore available information. Laws prohibit insurers from using race or sex in setting premiums, and many companies prefer to deny insurance to sick applicants, rather than to charge actuarially fair rates.[10]

Oddly enough, even if forecasts, available *before* patients enroll, are accurate enough to prevent market failure, the gradual acquisition of information by insurers about their customers *after* enrollment can create additional problems, since this information is not readily available to competitors. Such postenrollment information creates incentives for insurers to encourage or to force enrollees to drop coverage. The most obvious way to create such incentives is to provide poor service for costly conditions. ("You have an unusual disease. I'll do what I can for you, but, quite frankly, our plan doesn't do a very good job with it. You would do better with Dr. X, who is in the plan down the street.") This strategy works if patients are misinformed about the availability of such services when they decide in which plans to enroll, if they make systematic errors in processing available information, or if the complexity of the alternatives and contingencies makes an informed choice impossibly complex. For example, many studies document that people form incorrect judgments about low-probability events and that decisions are heavily influenced by framing.

Inferior Equilibrium

Even if insurance market outcomes are stable, they may be inferior, difficult, or impossible to dislodge. Peter Diamond presents an example in which an insurance market with a choice between two plans can produce results inferior to those when only one plan is available. Assume that there are two types of people, 1 and 2, and two insurance plans, A and B. Each plan is assumed to charge a single price for insurance coverage equal to average cost. *U* indicates the individual's evaluation of the benefits from enrolling in a plan; *C* indicates the cost to the plan of enrolling only people of a given type. The following matrix illustrates the problem:

Plan	Type 1	Type 2	Average cost of universal coverage
A	U = 23, C = 17	U = 20, C = 13	15
B	U = 8, C = 5	U = 7, C = 3	4

In this example, if two plans exist, persons of type 1 belong to plan A, the price of which is 17, leaving person 1 with a surplus of 6. At that price persons of type 2 choose plan B, which costs 3 and generates a utility surplus of 4. Neither type of person is tempted to change plans at the price they observe in the market. If universal coverage were imposed under plan A, however, the average-cost price would be 15, leaving people of type 1 with a surplus of 9 and people of type 2 with a surplus of 5, making both groups better off. Both the single-plan situation and the two-plan situation are stable equilibria. The two-plan situation, the one with the greater choice, is inferior for both parties.

Too much stress should not be placed on this example. It rests on asymmetrical information and the restriction to average cost pricing, characteristics that are common and important in health insurance but less important in most other markets. The introduction of additional plans intermediate between these two might break either or both of these equilibria. But it is not clear that any alternative equilibrium would be Pareto superior. In short, given these parameter values, the situation with choice could be unambiguously inferior to the situation without it.

Time Inconsistency

Standard economic analysis assumes that individuals' preferences are consistent over time. Consistency means that if $d_{it} > d_{jt}$, then $d_{is} > d_{js}$, where d_{kn} is a preference ranking of some situation k at time n, "$>$" means "is preferred to," and the relation between any two situations holds for all time periods. Of course, rankings may change if new information becomes available, but not otherwise. In general, future benefits and costs are discounted, so that early benefits are preferred to later benefits of the same instantaneous size and later costs are preferred to earlier costs. Exponential discounting is a necessary and sufficient condition for such time consistency (Strotz 1955).

Unfortunately, the experimental literature is replete with examples that violate consistency. If people are asked how much they would demand one month hence to forgo an immediate payment of $100, they typically name sums such as $110, $125, or even more, which imply annual interest rates enormously higher (214 percent, 1,355 percent, or even more, respectively) than actual yields at which people voluntarily save. If preferences are consistent, people would give the same answer when asked how much they would demand in thirteen months to forgo $100 in twelve months—the time interval is identical. In fact, most respondents state a much smaller premium to wait the extra month if they have to wait one year anyway. This example means that after twelve months, people find themselves locked into one-month contracts they would not voluntarily make at that time. Similar time inconsistency shows up with risk (Rachlin and Ranieri 1992). In these cases, people are offered $100 with certainty one month (or thirteen months) hence and asked what probability of $100 today (or twelve months hence) would leave one indifferent.[11] The important characteristic of these examples is that choices change even though preferences do not. One way of explaining such behavior is to posit that people use nonexponential discounting (Ainslie 1992; Laibson 1997).

Once again, it is important not to overinterpret such results. Although people reject enormously favorable odds in some circumstances, they continue to save and invest, and capital markets continue to function extremely well. The tendency to apply high discounts in short-term decisions raises the question of whether annual (or more frequent) shifts in insurance status are optimal, particularly given other research findings that suggest people do very poorly at handling low-probability events rationally.

Learning Curves

The existence of learning curves also influences the sustainability of competition and the performance of actual markets (Spence 1981). Learning curves can obstruct entry because they cause the long-run marginal costs of production to decline with total output. As a result, the profit-maximizing price for each company may be below current marginal cost. When learning is extremely fast or extremely slow, the barriers to entry are insignificant—in the former case because every company rapidly achieves whatever learning-curve economies are potentially available, and in the latter case because the cost reductions from learning are too small to matter much. But for intermediate rates of learning, early entrants can achieve production costs low enough to allow pricing strategies that make entry unprofitable for other companies. Exactly how an industry shakes out depends not only on the rate of learning, but also on the price elasticity of demand and the rate of growth of the market. Depending on the values of these parameters, the market may perform well or poorly relative to the lowest-cost ideal.

In health care, supply-side learning curves consist in being able to perform procedures more cheaply or more effectively as experience accumulates at scales relevant to total market demand. In this case, the learning curve may depend not only on total production, but also on the rate of production, because expertise and efficiency, once achieved, can atrophy if not maintained by continued high output. Both phenomena are well documented with respect to surgery, where cumulative experience and sustained higher rates of service are associated with improved outcomes and lower cost, although the evidence is less clear on the latter. Restrictions on the numbers of centers at which particular procedures are performed can lower cost and raise quality. This example clearly illustrates that regulation, public or private, to discourage new suppliers from entering the market holds the potential to raise welfare. For this reason, managed health plans that can focus their demands on high-quality, low-cost providers have an important potential advantage over unregulated systems, precisely because they can limit choice. A practical question is whether managed care plans sacrifice quality in the name of low cost, a clear agency problem. As is always the case, restrictions on entry carry a cost—the possibility that those suppliers who are initially in the market fail to introduce new methods (treatments) or technologies or become insensitive to customer (patient or insurer) preferences. How much restriction is desirable is a matter of facts and circumstances.

Paternalism

Diverse motivations underlie cash and in-kind assistance. The desire to redistribute income helps explain cash assistance and medical benefits for the poor. Concern about market failure may go some way toward explaining Medicare. But any list of justifications for programs such as Social Security and Medicare would be incomplete without acknowledging the dominant role of paternalism. These programs rest on a belief that many people would fail to make decisions in their own self-interest if left alone. They would discount the future too heavily and save too little. They would engage in psychological "denial"—the refusal to realistically appraise future risks, such as disability or illness—and fail to protect themselves adequately. They would base decisions on frivolous values or poor information. They would end up in a mess; the rest of us know it, and we are sure we would be so disturbed by that outcome that we willingly subject everyone, ourselves included, to the compulsions of taxes, mandatory annuitization, specified insurance benefits, and other restrictions on individual choice. None of these considerations requires Social Security or Medicare to take their current forms, but they do mean that free choice on how much to save and in what form to save is likely to leave many people—even those who are far from poor—poorly prepared when earnings cease or illness strikes.

Let me be clear—I come to praise paternalism, not to bury it. Standard economic analysis rests on assumptions that undermine any basis for paternalism, but these assumptions are false, whatever their value in advancing economic analysis.[12] Paternalism reflects an accurate judgment that private decisions produce consequences that no compassionate society is willing to tolerate. The practical questions, of course, are what forms the paternalism should take and whether the failures of individual decision making are more or less serious than the failings of collective decision making. Public choice theorists and empirical researchers have done everyone a great service by directing attention to analysis of the latter category of failings and their costs.

The Effects of Added Choice: Short and Long Run

At the start of 1997, Medicare faced both explosive growth in long-term spending and imminent insolvency in the Hospital Insurance Trust Fund. The Balanced Budget Act of 1997, together with systemwide slowdown in the growth of health care spending, reduced the first problem and temporarily solved the second. Projected growth in the overall cost of Medicare to 2035 as a share of GDP fell by about a quarter. Insolvency of the Hospital Insurance Trust Fund moved from 2002 to 2011. The 1997 legislation also marginally broadened the list of services that Medicare provides and, as described above, greatly expanded choice for Medicare enrollees. None of the projected savings reflected Medicare-specific effects of extending choice, which produced what I have called inflation-in-the-small. The legislated savings come mostly from reductions in reimbursement to providers (especially home care), reduced sharing in the costs of capital investment and education, and increased patient charges.

Although the growth of Medicare spending was reduced and insolvency of the Hospital Insurance Trust Fund delayed, large problems remained, as the Balanced Budget Act itself explicitly recognized, by calling for the creation of a bipartisan commission to propose fundamental long-term reforms. A major series of studies under the sponsorship of the National Academy of Social Insurance is addressing similar issues. What role should choice play in those reforms, and what restrictions on choice will give it the best chance to promote cost-effective health care services?

Benefit Coverage

The Medicare benefit package is far less complete than the standard benefit package of private insurance for the working-age population. It is, in fact, far less generous than the typical total benefit package for Medicare enrollees. All but 13 percent of enrollees enjoy supplemental wraparound coverage from employers, Medicaid, or personally financed Medigap insurance. The presence of this supplemental insurance has important consequences that are relevant to future reforms. First, Medigap insurance and employer wraparounds mute the intended demand-reducing effects of Medicare deductibles, copayments, and cost sharing. Supplemental insurance therefore raises Medicare program costs. Second, managed care alternatives to standard fee-for-service Medicare usually are able to provide some services other than those covered by Medicare (see table 2.1) for one or more of the reasons cited above—greater efficiency, favorable selection, stinting on care, or overly generous capitation. But each plan provides different services. Third, the diversity of benefit packages offered by managed care alternatives to traditional Medicare makes intelligent comparison shopping by Medicare patients extremely difficult even for health care economists, impossible for most Medicare beneficiaries, and a refined torture for those who are handicapped by mental or physical infirmities. Furthermore, benefit packages are a recognized instrument of risk selection. Offering sports medicine benefits, for example, is more appealing to the healthy enrollees than to those with chronic emphysema.

I believe that a necessary condition for well-functioning competition in Medicare is the establishment of a *uniform* and *expanded* benefit package that covers not only current Medicare benefits, but also many of those in wraparound benefits.[13] Uniformity is necessary because intelligent comparison of the costs of plans is impossible if benefit packages differ and benefits can be used to select low-cost patients. Uniformity also removes one tool of risk selection. Expanded benefits are necessary because the current package is so parsimonious that supplementation is inescapable and, as a practical matter, it would be impossible politically to deny people significant benefits to which they now have access. Furthermore, widespread use of supplemental benefits distorts incentives within the basic plan. An expanded package would certainly include effective catastrophic coverage, drug benefits, and reduced cost sharing.

Payments

The *average* Medicare payment on behalf of all people in a given health care market would equal some fraction of the average cost that health plans operating in that market incur in providing the basic package. The determination of the fraction would be the device by which elected officials would control the division of cost of health care for Medicare enrollees between the enrollees themselves and active workers or other taxpayers. Enrollees would be responsible for the balance of premium costs, which would vary from plan to plan. The *actual* payment made to each plan on behalf of *each* enrollee should probably be a blend of a capitation payment determined prospectively and a service payment determined retrospectively. The reason for partial retrospective payments is that no plausible risk-adjustment algorithm can account for significant variation in health costs among patients that is unpredictable *ex ante* but becomes predictable *ex post*, creating incentives for health plans to try to drive away high-cost patients or to stint on care. A variety of devices exists to deal with this problem, including partial fee-for-service payments on a patient-by-patient basis, reinsurance, or case-mix adjustments. It might prove desirable to carve out particular services to be provided by separate providers under separate payment arrangements in order to minimize the need for payments to offset outlier costs that bedevil all but very large plans.[14] The practical question with respect to such mixed plans is whether the information costs and bureaucratic burdens associated with collecting the information and applying it to plan administration would outweigh any benefits. Only experimentation can settle that question.

All Medicare enrollees would face the same out-of-pocket charge for a given plan. Uniform pricing sacrifices some potential gains from the incentive effects of price variation (encouraging exercise or promoting moderate alcoholic consumption, for example). Of course, the standard plans could include limited copayments and coinsurance to discourage frivolous demands. The reason for uniform charges is that the major sources of variability in demands for care arise from factors that are beyond the control of the patient—genetic inheritance, race, sex, age, prior work history, accidents, and the random incidence of illness and debility. Apart from possible discounts for readily identified behaviors (not smoking, for example), price differentials based on such factors would capriciously penalize and reward people. I am arguing that such variations in medical use should be averaged over the population.

While plans might offer supplementary benefits, both the nature of such benefits and the price charged for them should be regulated to make sure that the price incorporates any extra cost or savings that the supplemental benefits induce in the basic plan. Such regulation is also necessary to minimize the use of supplemental benefits as an instrument of risk selection.

Criticisms

The force of the preceding argument is that unfettered individual choice and unregulated business practices in health care will make competition inefficient. A uniform benefit package with limited and regulated supplementation is necessary to give competition the greatest chance to encourage efficient delivery of health care. Such limits are open to criticism on a number of grounds.

The first is that the approach to benefits is a classical example of "one size fits all." This criticism is, I believe, mindless nonsense in this case. The utility of medical care comes from the availability of care appropriate to medical problems, not from varying insurance contract language. A benefit package that covers the services that most people demand does not constrain them to uniform services. On the contrary, it assures each person access to diverse treatment tailored to his or her specific needs and wants. Individuals would still be free to choose such differing delivery modes as full closed-panel HMOs, point-of-service plans, PPOs, and fee-for-service delivery, provided that they pay out-of-pocket for the extra costs of relatively expensive systems.

The second criticism is that this approach would be expensive and cumbersome to administer. On this score, the verdict is "guilty as charged, but with extenuating circumstances." Collecting data necessary to both risk-adjust and to make some form of retrospective payment would be a major burden. Demonstrations need to be run to evaluate what those costs would be. These costs can be justified only because managed competition cannot function without risk adjustment and the best possible risk-adjustment algorithms still will leave such profit so that in trying to select patients, the efficiency gains from competition will be threatened.

It is unclear whether the benefits of full managed competition will outweigh the costs of making it work. But the alternative is not a return to traditional fee-for-service Medicare. The cost of unrestricted moral hazard operating in a field as technologically dynamic as medicine is insupportable. Regulation, meaning limits on free choice, is inescapable and desirable.

We Can Get There from Here, but It Is Harder Now

I have argued that making competition work in Medicare requires a more generous and more uniform benefit structure than the current Medicare system contains, in combination with its various supplements. This step will boost budget costs of Medicare, but if successful, it will lower total medical spending adjusted for the quality of care. The reforms of Medicare contained in the Balanced Budget Act of 1997 will make achievement of this goal more difficult. The reason is that profits from risk selection and any gains from improved efficiency as patients shift into one form or another of managed care are likely to lead to a proliferation of diverse benefits, possibly more generous than would be contained in a liberalized, uniform package. The extra benefits will reflect the fact that the method of paying managed care is tied to fee-for-service costs, which are likely to rise if managed care plans continue to achieve favorable selection. The result is likely to be a crazy quilt of benefits that will pose vexing political problems for future Congresses bent on helping competition work effectively.

Notes

1. All quotations are from Harris Meyer (1997).

2. Strictly speaking, they have had access to three kinds of alternatives to traditional fee-for-service Medicare: so-called *risk* plans, which accept a per capita payment from the Health Care Financing Administration and have been authorized since 1982; *cost* plans, first authorized in 1972, which receive a prospective fee based on plan costs; and *prepayment* plans, first authorized by the original legislation creating Medicare, which operate like cost plans but do not cover Part A services.

3. The Kaiser Medicare Policy Project, p. 73, figure 33.

4. When risk contracting became feasible, the chief executive of a major managed care plan with whom I had a private conversation looked forward gleefully to marketing to the elderly. "Here is what we will do," he said. "We will sponsor dances, invite the elderly, and make our sales pitch at about 11 P.M."

5. For a description of these changes, see Moon, Gage, and Evans (1998).

6. Starting in 2002 enrollees in Medicare + Choice options will be able, as a rule, to return to traditional Medicare during the first six months of the year. Beginning in 2003 enrollees will be permitted to leave their "choice" plans during the first three months of the year and will be locked in for the remainder of the year.

7. Some algorithms turn out to solve such problems in practice—the simplex algorithm for linear programming, for example—although they are not guaranteed to work.

8. For a particularly beguiling example of the first-order effects of simple labeling, it is hard to beat the experiment reported by Ross and Ward (1996). In this experiment, Stanford proctors were instructed to select two groups of students based on the proctors' judgments about which residents would be most likely to cooperate and which most likely to defect in a prisoners' dilemma game. The likely cooperators and defectors were each split in two. Two new groups were formed, each consisting half of likely cooperators and half of likely defectors. Each of the new groups played games with identical payoff matrices. The only difference was the name the experimenters assigned to the games. One was called the Wall Street Game and the other was called the Community Game. In each group, the likely cooperators and the likely defectors performed almost identically, suggesting that the judgments of the proctors about who would cooperate and who would defect were worthless. But 65 percent of those playing the Com-

munity Game cooperated, while only 30 percent of those playing the Wall Street Game cooperated. For an almost endless list of such violations of the canons of rational decision making, see Nisbett and Ross (1980), Ross and Nisbett (1991), Camerer (1995), and Rabin (1998).

9. For some notable exceptions, see Akerlof and Yellin (1994); Akerlof and Kranton (1998); Kuran (1995); and Glaeser, Sacerdote and Scheinkman (1996).

10. The Kennedy-Kassebaum Bill requires insurance companies to sell insurance to workers who change jobs but does not stipulate rules for setting premiums, some of which are as much as six times normal rates. As this paper is being written, members of Congress are threatening legislation to prevent insurers from setting premiums the insurers deem necessary to offer such coverage (Pear 1998).

11. Good introductions to such "anomalies" are Rabin (1998), Loewenstein and Prelec (1992), Camerer (1995), and, more generally, the series of columns in the *Journal of Economic Perspectives* by Richard Thaler.

12. It is true, of course, that most behaviors can be explained within traditional models with sufficiently imaginative adjustments. While this observation is true, it is not a sign of strength, as powerful theories must be refutable. As Herbert Simon (1986) points out, "Neoclassical theory, as usually applied, is an exceedingly weak theory, as shown by the difficulty of finding sets of facts, actual or hypothetical, that cannot be rationalized and made consistent with it."

13. Alain Enthoven and Richard Kronick (1989), strong advocates of managed competition, have placed great emphasis on the need for a standard benefit package and other regulatory interventions on the grounds that competition would fail without them.

14. For a thorough explanation of these issues, a description of devices that have been developed to deal with them, and a call for extensive research before final decisions are made, see National Academy of Social Insurance (1998).

References

Aaron, Henry. 1994. "Distinguished Lecture on Economics in Government: Public Policy, Values, and Consciousness," *Journal of Economic Perspectives* 8 (2).

Ainslie, George. 1992. *Picoeconomics*. Cambridge: Cambridge University Press.

Akerlof, George A. 1984. *An Economic Theorist's Book of Tales*. Cambridge: Cambridge University Press.

Akerlof, George, and Rachel Kranton. 1999. "Economics and Identity." Manuscript.

Akerlof, George, and Janet Yellin. 1994. "Gang Behavior, Law Enforcement, and Community Values." In *Values and Public Policy*, edited by Henry J. Aaron, Thomas E. Mann, and Timothy Taylor. Washington, D.C.: Brookings Institution.

American Association of Health Plans. 1998. Policy Brief 1/3-98. *The Medicare Risk Contracting Program: Facts and Figures: November 1997.*

Becker, Gary. 1996. *The Economic Way of Looking at Behavior: The Nobel Lecture*. Hoover Institution. Stanford: Stanford University.

Camerer, Colin. 1995. "Individual Decision Making." In *The Handbook of Experimental Economics*, edited by John H. Kagel and Alvin E. Roth. Princeton: Princeton University Press, pp. 587–703.

Diamond, Peter. 1992. "Organizing the Health Insurance Market." *Econometrica* 60 (6): 1,233–54.

Enthoven, Alain, and Richard Kronick. 1989. "A Consumer-Choice Health Plan for the 1990s: Universal Health Insurance in a System Designed to Promote Quality and Economy." *New England Journal of Medicine* 320: 29–37, 94–101.

Glaeser, Edward, Bruce Sacerdote, and José Scheinkman. 1996. "Crime and Social Interactions." *The Quarterly Journal of Economics* 111 (2): 507–48.

Komisar, Harriet L., James A. Reuter, Judith Feder, and Patricia Neuman. 1997. *Medicare Chart Book*. Menlo Park, Calif.: Henry J. Kaiser Foundation.

Kuran, Timur. 1995. *Private Truths, Public Lies: The Social Consequences of Preference Falsification*. Cambridge: Harvard University Press.

Laibson, David. 1997. "Golden Eggs and Hyperbolic Discounting." *Quarterly Journal of Economics* 112 (2): 443–77.

LeRoy, Lauren, Jack Hoadley, and Katie Merrell. 1997. *Medicare Risk-Plan Participation and Enrollment: A Chart Book*. Washington, D.C.: Medicare Payment Advisory Commission.

Loewenstein, George, and Drazen Prelec. 1992. "Anomalies in Intertemporal Choice: Evidence and Interpretation." In *Choice over Time*, edited by George Loewenstein and Jon Elster. New York: Russell Sage Foundation, pp. 119–47.

Meyer, Harris. 1997. "The Medicare Mall: Will Washington Like What It Built?" *Hospitals and Health Networks* 71 (no. 23, 5 December): 26–32.

Moon, Marilyn, Barbara Gage, and Alison Evans. 1998. *An Examination of Key Medicare Provisions in the Balanced Budget Act of 1997*. New York: Commonwealth Fund.

National Academy of Social Insurance (NASI). 1998. *Structuring Medicare Choices*, Final Report of the Study Panel on Capitation and Costs, Washington, D.C.

Nisbett, Richard, and Lee Ross. 1980. *Human Inference: Strategies and Shortcomings of Social Judgment*. New York: Prentice-Hall.

Oaksford, M., and N. Chater. 1993. "Reasoning Theories and Bounded Rationality." In *Rationality: Psychological and Philosophical Perspectives,* edited by K. I. Manktelow and D. E. Over. New York: Routledge, pp. 31–60.

Pear, Robert. 1998. "High Rates Hobble Law to Guarantee Health Insurance." *New York Times* (17 March), p. 1.

Rabin, Mathew. 1998. "Psychology and Economics." *Journal of Economic Literature* 36 (1): 11–46.

Rachlin, Howard, and Andres Raineri. 1992. "Irrationality, Impulsiveness, and Selfishness as Discount Reversal Effects." In *Choice over Time*, edited by George Loewenstein and Jon Elster. New York: Russell Sage, pp. 93–118.

Ross, Lee, and Richard Nisbett. 1991. *The Person and the Situation*. Philadelphia: Temple University Press.

Ross, Lee, and Andrew Ward. 1996. "Naive Realism in Everyday Life: Implications for Social Conflict and Misunderstanding." In *Values and Knowledge*, edited by T. Brown, E. Reed, and E. Turiel. Hillsdale, N.J.: Erlbaum, pp. 103–135.

Simon, Herbert A. 1986. "Rationality in Psychology and Economics." *Journal of Business* 59 (4, pt. 2): S209–S224.

Spence, Michael. 1981. "The Learning Curve and Competition." *The Bell Journal of Economics* 12 (1): 49–70.

Stiglitz, Joseph E., and Michael Rothschild. 1976. "Equilibrium in Competitive Insurance Markets: An Essay on the Economics of Imperfect Information." *Quarterly Journal of Economics* 90: 629–49.

Strotz, Robert. 1955. "Myopia and Inconsistency in Dynamic Utility Maximization." *Review of Economic Studies* 23: 165–80.

Chapter Three

Should Medicare Be Less Generous to Higher-Income Beneficiaries?

Mark V. Pauly

Introduction

The Medicare program was created to help retired people afford adequate medical care. In the first quarter of the next century, achievement of this objective is now threatened by the rising cost of the program and the falling growth rate of the working-age tax base, which supports over 90 percent of the program's cost. In the face of this difficult future, it is both necessary and desirable to determine whether the program can be restructured in a way that allows its goals to continue to be met under a financing system that is less politically and economically threatened. One way to do so that will improve both equity and efficiency is a reduction in the generosity of Medicare's contribution toward the health insurance purchases of higher-income or higher-wealth beneficiaries.

There have been some surprising changes in the retired population, in the nature of medical care services, and in the focus of health policy since Medicare was enacted in 1965. Modifying the program to fit these changes, possibly desirable in any case, can produce necessary improvements.

The change in the over-65 population that is noteworthy is the increased numbers of moderate- and higher-income (and higher-wealth)

Mark V. Pauly, Ph.D., is the Bendheim Professor; chair and professor of the Health Care Systems Department; vice dean and director of doctoral programs, at the Wharton School, University of Pennsylvania.

households in this population. It is commonplace to remark that when Medicare was passed, being old was virtually synonymous with being poor. Now the proportion of households below the poverty line is lower in this age group than for any other in the population. Less frequently noticed is that this improvement actually has two dimensions. A large part of this shift resulted from the spread and enhancement of Social Security, which raised many elderly households to income levels above—but only slightly above—the poverty line. The less noticed phenomenon is the increase as well in the proportion of the elderly population with incomes comfortably above the poverty line.

At present, well-to-do elders receive exactly the same tax-supported coverage and pay the same premiums as do those with incomes just above the poverty line. In contrast, Social Security benefits are lower for higher-income elders. Only those so poor as to be on Medicaid will pay less or get more. In this chapter, I will explore the rationales and methods for modifying the Medicare program to treat the well-off segment of the population differently. My primary motive for doing so, however, is not based on considerations of equity, intergenerational redistribution, or trust-fund posturing. Rather, I want to argue that current patterns of Medicare coverage are *inefficient* because the current level of public insurance is excessively generous for the well-off. Their insurance is more generous, and more costly, even after adjusting for health status, than for their under-65 counterparts (even though the latter receive partial tax subsidies). Moreover, I will argue that this inefficiency is compounded, for the great majority of this population, by the way in which supplemental Medigap coverage is treated. Finally, even if the shift to Medicare managed care continues, these problems, I argue, may still remain.

I will recommend that, for this subpopulation, Medicare be converted to an income- and wealth-related *defined contribution or voucher* program, a step that will improve efficiency in the medical insurance market while it reduces the future burden of Medicare on workers and makes Medicare more similar to other subsidy programs. I emphasize that in order to achieve the objective of improved efficiency, it will be necessary to make major (not marginal) changes in subsidy levels and required coverage.

A second change since the passage of Medicare has been the change in the nature of the medical services product. Changes in technology have brought about changes in medical services, which represent improvements in quality but at a substantially higher cost. These changes, as far as we can tell, have occurred in medical services for the Medicare population at about the same rate as in services for the rest of the population. Normative judgments are trickier here, since it is far from clear what citizens should expect from the Medicare program in terms of trends for quality improvement. I will argue, however, that there need be no social commitment to provide *higher* quality than at present to higher-income/higher-wealth Medicare beneficiaries. It may be both equitable and efficient for households with high levels of lifetime income to finance their own improved quality; doing so may limit either inequity (higher Medicare quality than for the rest of the population) or inefficiency (higher quality than is justified by the cost).

We *can* today guarantee state-of-the-art medicine to all of the elderly in 2020 with almost no increase in tax rates. However, the quality that can be provided by such financing will be nearer to 1998 state-of-the-art than to the forecasted 2020 version. The key normative question then is what level of publicly financed access to improvements in health are owed future cohorts of elders, especially nonpoor elders, compared to today's beneficiaries. This is not, then, a question of redistribution of a fixed amount of well-being within or across generations; it is an issue of who should pay for and who should receive the increase in the size of the health and survival pie.

Finally, at the broader level of policy, Medicare should be blended more smoothly with other subsidy programs. More ambitiously, all such programs might be integrated into a single scheme to subsidize and ensure universal coverage, regardless of age. For reasons already hinted at, the institutional arrangement of an age-related social insurance program may be increasingly anachronistic in a changing world.

Data on Medicare and the Economy

Medicare was passed to offer enhanced insurance to those over 65. Improved insurance coverage makes two changes in those it affects. It reduces the variation in out-of-pocket medical care spending, thereby reducing as well the variation in the amount of income or wealth that can be spent on other things. It also increases the amount and type of medical care consumed because of the well-known and well-established "moral hazard" associated with insurance when the insurer cannot costlessly observe the insured's severity of illness (Pauly 1971).

The social objectives of Medicare were better protection against risk *and* facilitation of higher rates of use of medical services. The legislative history makes it clear that the low levels of both such factors among the 1965 elderly were viewed to be the problem. Better risk protection for all was one goal. The other was to generate *more* moral hazard among those elders thought previously to be using inappropriately low amounts and qualities of care. Since 1965, however, the proportion of elders with family incomes above the poverty line has increased. Table 3.1 shows the dramatic change in the level and distribution of income among elderly households between 1967, a year after the enactment of Medicare, and 1996. Not only did the proportion in poverty drop from 29 percent to 9 percent, but the proportion with incomes above 200 percent of the poverty line rose from 37 percent to 60 percent of households. The proportion above 400 percent of the poverty line, which is usually interpreted as upper-middle income, doubled from 12 percent to 24 percent of the elderly.

What impact does Medicare coverage have on the reasonably well-off population? In reality, most research has concentrated on poor and near-poor elders; little is known about the important and growing well-off segment of the population. In particular, we do not know whether this population might purchase private insurance if Medicare did not exist, whether it might use less care, and whether its health would be affected. In what follows, I briefly review the fragmentary theory and evidence applying to this question.

Table 3.1 Percent Distribution of Elderly by Family Income as Percentage of Poverty Line

Income/Poverty Level	**1968**	**1997**
< 100%	28.6%	9.1%
< 200	34.3%	30.6%
< 300	16.3%	21.9%
< 400	9.3%	13.9%
< 500	4.9%	8.5%
500+	6.6%	15.9%

SOURCE: Author's tabulation from Current Population Survey.

We know in theory one effect that higher wealth should have on the use of care for consumers: Given some illness level and the same level of insurance coverage, the higher-wealth group will choose higher levels of care. They may choose more quality, and they surely will also choose more costly care. The relevant (risk-adjusted) income elasticity of quantity demanded appears to be about 0.2 (Phelps 1997, 151); by this calculation, a family with $40,000 a year income would be expected to demand 40 percent more care, given the level of health, than a family with a $10,000 income. Moreover, spending appears to increase more than physical quantity, as higher-priced sources of care are used. In addition, there is evidence as well that these higher levels of spending improve survival—which means that higher-income persons live more years in which they receive Medicare benefits (Hadley 1982; Newhouse et al. 1993).

What about a possible effect of moral hazard, given income? Several pieces of empirical evidence support the theoretical expectations that even higher-income people use more care the more generously it is covered. Most rigorously, we know from the Rand Health Insurance Experiment that higher levels of insurance coverage unequivocally encourage greater use and higher expenditures for all types of care (Newhouse et al., 1993). We also know that this effect is equally strong for higher-income households as for lower-income ones, although richer households start at high levels of use. They increase their spending as coverage becomes more generous. While the experiment did not cover people with very high incomes, those with no insurance, or the elderly, one may expect these general patterns to extend to them.

At the level of aggregate data, the evidence is strong that higher-income elderly have higher medical care spending over their period of Medicare eligibility (McClellan and Skinner 1997). There are at least two indirect causes for this phenomenon: higher lifetime income leads to better health and longevity, largely for reasons unrelated to access to medical care. In addition, higher-income elderly are more likely to buy or obtain supplemental coverage (Medigap), which is known to stimulate spending. Indeed, it is the effect of such supplemental coverage that provides the strongest nonexperimental evidence for moral hazard. To complete the argument about rates of use, we would like direct evidence that, controlling for health status and insurance coverage, higher-income people who still pay something out-of-pocket use more care than lower-income people.

In addition to the positive effect of income on demand given insurance coverage, there is also strong evidence that higher income leads to purchase of more generous levels of insurance coverage, even in the absence of the tax subsidy. Specifically, Medicare beneficiaries with incomes just above the limit for Medicaid eligibility are much less likely to purchase or obtain supplementary coverage that those with higher incomes. In short, the willingness to pay both for care and coverage (at a given price) rises with income.

Goals for Medicare and the Economy

How do we judge these facts? A classic social insurance model would impose taxes related positively to a person's wages (not income) below some target age; then taxes could turn negative (become subsidies) after that age.[1] In the case of Social Security, higher working-age tax contributions were intended to mean somewhat higher benefits, since the level of benefits is explicitly tied to earning levels in covered employment. For Medicare, the social purpose was and is more confused. Since its inception, all Medicare beneficiaries have been eligible for exactly the same nominal insurance coverage. However, the after-the-fact distribution of benefits is far from equal. Higher-income persons make more use of the insurance, so much so that, according to some estimates, Medicare actually redistributes to higher-income households on a lifetime basis (McClellan and Skinner 1997), although greater redistribution to those who suffer the fate of living too long may not be so unfair. Alternatively, one may view higher lifetime Medicare spending as only a symptom of the central problem of maldistribution of life years: compared to the rest of us, there are more life years for the well-to-do (and thin physiques as well).

Is the purpose of Medicare to produce or support such a pattern of inequality? The history of the program does not suggest so. The benefit was supposed to be highly egalitarian. The higher benefits per period and over their lifetime for higher-income persons were surely unintended consequences.

Purely on equity or "social design" grounds, then, one might propose some adjustment in the current Medicare program, an adjustment that would have the well-to-do pay more. Not only would this be fairer, but it would help to preserve the "solvency" of the program at constant payroll tax rates. However, the key question is how this larger contribution might be extracted. But how far should we go?

Efficient Consumption

The optimal pattern of care—and therefore the optimal pattern of user prices and subsidies—depends on both the effect of income on private demand given illness (which I will henceforth assume is positive and large enough to matter) and the social goal. Modeling the objectives of Medicare (or any other social program) is obviously an essay in informed speculation; the most we can hope for is plausibility (subject to the ultimate test of political acceptability).

I have explored this question some time ago (and actually considered its application to then newly passed Medicare) (Pauly 1971). Here I will summarize and add to that discussion. One way to model social objectives is to assume that, in addition to individuals' private demands for care for themselves, many citizens also attach real value to (and have demand for) medical care to be provided to others. This motivation is most obviously present in the case of contagious disease (Phelps 1997), but the much more important case is one based on feelings of concern about treatable but untreated illness—in economic jargon, an "altruistic externality."

We can describe this social demand in per beneficiary terms by postulating a community marginal valuation or demand curve D_c. This curve shows, for a representative Medicare beneficiary with the average expectation of illness, what values the rest of the community would place on additional medical care for him or her. The first unit of care would be of high (though not infinite) value, but then marginal values would decline. We do not know empirically the slope or elasticity of this curve, although some studies based on Medicaid indicate that the elasticity is neither infinite nor zero.

For purpose of illustration, I will initially follow the suggestion of Paul Feldstein (1988, 527–29) and suppose that the curve is close to perfectly inelastic. This is equivalent to describing the social motivation as if there were consensus on a unique amount of "needed" or "appropriate" care, in the sense that society feels terrible if the person uses less than the targeted amount but perceives no benefit whatsoever if he or she uses more than the targeted amount. In this case in figure 3.1, the

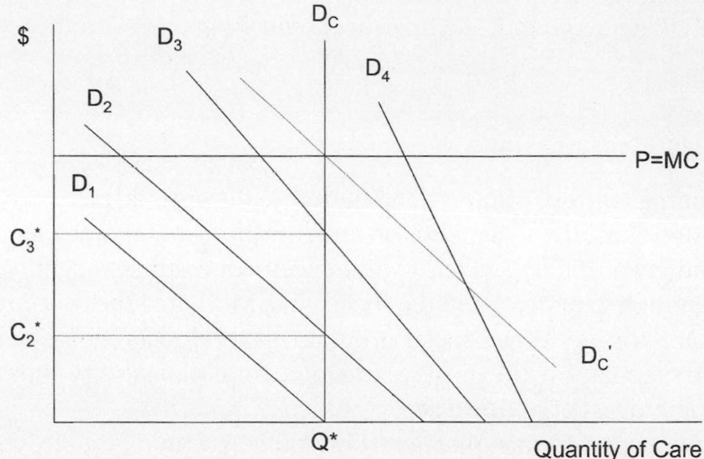

Figure 3.1 Private and Collective Demand for Medical Care

community demand curve D_c is nearly vertical at some optimal expected quantity per capita Q^*. The four demand curves are for different income groups, in ascending order. I assume that demands differ only by income. The implication is obvious: To achieve Q^*, the lowest-income groups should get free care, the two middle groups should pay some positive coinsurance C_2^* or C_3^*, and the richest group needs no insurance at all. If instead the D_c demand curve is as D_c', the optimal quantities (not shown) will increase with income (but become more equal than with no subsidy). However, the qualitative pattern of optimal cost sharing will be the same.

The implication of this analysis for elders at different income levels is obvious but profound. In some fashion, we need to ensure that group 1 receives full coverage insurance and that groups 2 and 3 get some but only partial coverage; for group 4, there is no need to assure or mandate any level of coverage. Of course, if this last group would choose to buy coverage on its own, no social harm is done, as long as it pays the full cost itself. Moreover, above some cutoff-income level at which the subsidy is ended, the desired (and therefore socially optimal) level of coverage might rise with income. Hence, the efficient pattern of coverage might be V shaped: high coverage for the poor, declining with incomes as incomes rise but a subsidy is still offered, and then rising after the subsidy is ended.

Comparison with Other Income-Related Schemes

The method usually suggested for reducing the burden of tax financing of Medicare by having the rich pay more is to increase the premium contribution of high-income elderly. Such an idea flourished briefly as part of the Medicare reform debate, tempting moderate Democrats as well as Republicans (Reischauer 1997a). Another proposal was to increase the Part A deductible modestly for higher-income beneficiaries. This idea also flared, even more briefly, during the reform debate and faded instantly.

I have something more sweeping and more dramatic in mind than either increased income-related premiums or reduced income-related Medicare coverage. Rather than just increase the deductible from conventional Medicare for higher-income beneficiaries, I envision a cut, severe at the highest income levels, in the dollar amount of Medicare payment on behalf of those beneficiaries—a cut that will take effect whether they choose to obtain insurance through conventional Medicare, managed care, or some other substitute. Medicare will take the form of a defined contribution (as it is already doing), but it should be an *income-related* defined contribution. At the same time, I also envision greatly reducing the generosity of the coverage the better-off elderly are required to buy in order to receive the subsidy that remains. For this minimum coverage limit, setting a maximum deductible (for example, 10 percent of income or wealth) would be one method of specification.

The precise numbers to be specified represent political choice, but here is an illustration of what I have in mind: Under current law, when I retire I can expect to receive from Medicare a subsidy or credit toward health insurance of approximately $5,000. Suppose that my retirement income will be $60,000 per year and that the fair premium for conventional Medicare coverage with a $6,000 deductible was $2,000. This is judged to be adequate coverage for someone as well-off in retirement as I will be. Finally, suppose that the subsidy or credit judged to be fair for my income level was $1,200. Then I would be required to buy a policy with a deductible no greater than $6,000 and therefore pay at least $800.

Note that this approach reduces cost to under-65 taxpayers in two ways. I am required to pay a premium for the obligatory or statutory coverage, and I am required to pay additionally, either out-of-pocket or through supplementary coverage, for expenses below the statutory deductible.

One final but important descriptive point: It is probable (and not necessarily undesirable, as we shall see below) that some high-income people may want to buy more generous coverage than the minimum amount—only the very wealthiest can afford to be uninsured. Purchase of Medigap coverage defeats the cost-containment effects of higher patient cost sharing so, critics say, why bother? Technically, no inefficiency in the insurance market would be created if the highest-income group were subsidized to buy the same level of coverage they would buy on their own. But the subsidy would be totally unnecessary and does cause the distortions associated with tax-financed payments. At all other income levels, however, the observation that in an otherwise efficiently functioning insurance market and at a given level of subsidy, people might choose to supplement the socially chosen basic catastrophic coverage has an important implication: it means that the final level of subsidy is too high.[2] If people are paying for additional coverage entirely with their own money, the subsidy is unnecessarily large. *The subsidy should be cut until the level of coverage falls to the optimal level or until the subsidy is eliminated, whichever comes first.* If (contrary to my assumption) people varied by risk aversion or taste for medical care, one might accept supplementation by part of the population as administrative simplification.

However, the current situation in which 70 percent of elderly obtain supplemental private coverage to Medicare does not provide definitive evidence on the demand for coverage in an efficiently functioning market. There is currently a serious distortion. People who buy Medigap policies definitely make greater use of conventional Medicare but pay nothing additional for it; effectively, there is currently a substantial cross-subsidy to Medigap coverage, which serves only to distort choices and raise costs. In the ideal system I am describing, people should either be required to purchase all their coverage from a single source or else pay higher premiums for basic coverage if they supplement it.

Finally, there is strong evidence that moderate-income people do economize on insurance purchases when those purchases are not heavily subsidized. For example, if Medicare's contribution to insurance was reduced, the well-off might choose not only less generous fee-for-service insurance but also more aggressive HMOs and ones offering fewer luxury benefits (Pauly 1996). In all of these cases, there is at least the opportunity to do more than just redistribute by making the better-off pay more. There are allocative effects as well, and they operate in the direction of reducing total spending. Of course, once spending at the margin is private rather than public, it will have only an indirect effect on Medicare's future.

The more thoroughgoing approach outlined here helps to avoid some of the objections raised to the Senate Finance Committee's proposal for income-related deductibles (Reischauer 1997a 1997b). First, the "income-relatedness" could be administered relatively easily through the income tax system. Rather than trying to base payment *ex ante* on current income, one could make payment based on estimated income, and then adjusted overpayment or underpayment later as part of the household's income tax. Ideally, wealth or consumption, not current realized income, should govern the extent of subsidy. Basing the subsidy on consumption would be the best way to implement this proposal. Then the person whose income is artificially inflated because of capital gains in one year would not need to have any adjustment made, since consumption is unlikely to fluctuate much. The household whose income falls because of a post-65 retirement of a family member would need an adjustment only in the unlikely event that consumption took a big drop as well.

More importantly, my proposal would not be limited to the richest 5 percent of elders (as the Senate one was) but would be applied to a large fraction of all elderly, perhaps to the 25 percent with incomes more than four times the poverty line. Even for those this well-off, it is incorrect to argue that they "are not likely to cut back on their use of services because they [are] not constrained budgetarily" (Reischauer 1997b)—given the Rand results, which (while not extending to the very wealthy) displayed no sign that the effect of cost sharing was starting to fall as income and wealth rose. The well-off might not have to cut back, but they do cut back (as do those at lower incomes) as the relative price increases.

Money and Managed Care

I have argued that the better-off should be less heavily subsidized in the purchase of conventional insurance coverage. For the 85 percent of Medicare beneficiaries currently using traditional indemnity insurance, this argument will be highly relevant. But what about the small (but growing) minority who use managed care? What is the socially efficient amount, type, and (most importantly) cost of coverage for them?

Surprisingly, there is very little evidence on differences in the types of managed care chosen by people at different income levels, although there is evidence that beyond some moderate income level, managed care is an inferior good. Choice of managed care modifications, such as point-of-service plans or wider networks, does seem positively related to income. In short, though we have yet to obtain fully definitive evidence, there is reason to believe that the choice of additional costly managed care benefits would be positively related to income.

In contrast to this reasonably assured conclusion, it is much less clear what the social optimum would be. For lower-income people, the optimum is presumably a reasonably prudent managed care plan with near-zero cost sharing. As income increases, it is reasonably clear that the optimum will not be much more generous. Perhaps the level of out-of-pocket payment and limits on provider choice need be no different than for the lower-income people; in such a case, the credit can be uniform and still be efficient. More generally, without knowing how (or whether) income still affects the use rate within a given managed care plan, we will not know the optimal pattern of strictness of coverage. But we can still conclude that the minimum subsidy needed to assure purchase of the minimally acceptable managed care plan should decline with income.

How Much More Is Enough?

Reducing the amount to be financed for higher-income elders will therefore reduce the aggregate burden of Medicare in the future. It would probably be politically best and morally fairest to phase in reductions in payments for these populations gradually. Doing so can cut the growth rate in Medicare spending dramatically and reduce the tax rate needed for spending at any date in the future.

However, even such a dramatic change in eligibility may not be enough to preserve the kind of Medicare spending growth that we have had in the past and still expect into the future. But does the social insurance program need to support that level of spending?

The key fact for this discussion is that the rise in Medicare spending per beneficiary over time has been primarily due to *higher levels of ben-*

eficial but costly technology. Just as with under-65 spending growth, there have also been periods when input prices for medical services have run ahead of wages and factor prices in the economy; but this pattern has been much less consistent, and, in any case, such "relative price" growth surely accounts for less than half of the real growth in expenditures per beneficiary (Pauly 1995). Moreover, as we look into the future, there is less reason to expect this pattern to continue, a topic I will discuss below.

Here are some approximate numbers that illustrate the importance of technical change in Medicare's future. The population of workers is projected to grow (under the intermediate assumption of the Social Security actuaries) at about 0.5 percent per year, while the elderly population is projected to have about a 2 percent growth rate. Taxes that are proportional to wages will therefore be able to continue to pay the same real dollar benefit per elderly person only if real taxable wages per worker grow at about a 1.5 percent rate (Board of Trustees 1997). Such a rate has occurred at some time periods since 1945, although not recently. The main conclusion, even so, is that current tax rates on wages (explicit for Part A, implicit for Part B) are sufficient or nearly sufficient to maintain future benefits at current levels in real terms, even with demographic changes. If the current high levels of worker wage growth should continue, or if fertility should rise soon, the possibility of constant tax rates would be enhanced. However, it will be impossible to maintain those tax rates if benefits are to rise in real terms.

Consider then someone expecting to go on Medicare in 2020 and to be at a relatively high-income or -wealth level. If tax rates are not increased, that person could receive a contribution from the social insurance system upon retiring that would allow purchase of insurance providing benefits adequate to purchase services with 1998 technology. If such a payment policy was announced, those persons who wanted to be able to obtain more costly technology in 2020 would presumably save privately (using the private market) to build up adequate wealth to pay for whatever additional technology they desired.

Who Gets What Type of Technology?

The issue of technology pushes us back to the murky territory of social objectives. For very low-income elderly, presumably government subsidies, not private savings, would be responsible for determining access to technology. In effect, for this population, society positively chooses how much of the new technology it wishes to make available. We might well decide to pay for new technology for this group. For higher-income elderly, if some do not choose costly but beneficial new technology, the observation that they could have saved to obtain it but choose not to do so might lead to acceptance of inequality. However, if new technology is a normal good, this group should choose to have reasonably good access, too. The main problem would arise for the middle group, those of moderate incomes, who might have purchased the new technology through insurance before they retired but might then find themselves unable or unwilling to purchase it afterward. These observations serve to focus on what is in a sense the fundamental Medicare dilemma. A group of people with moderate lifetime incomes wants a type of care when they retire that they cannot pay for and no one can afford to purchase for them.

We cannot settle this problem directly, but here are some considerations that may be relevant. First, under-65 insureds might also demand lower levels of new technology because most of them are now covered by managed care. There is some evidence that managed care plans are less likely to adopt new technology than are (or were) conventional plans. However, the evidence on this point is far from conclusive at present. Second, whether it is socially objectionable for some elderly to have less access to technology than some people under 65 depends on our understanding of the reason of growth in under-65 spending. Conventional insurance, fostered by the tax subsidy, surely lead to *levels* of spending for this population being excessive (because of moral hazard), and there is some evidence that moral hazard is the cause of much of the growth in spending (Peden and Freedland 1995). So if the growth in spending among the under-65 population in the future is thought to be likely to remain high because of moral hazard, or bad incentives generally, those who think that such growth is wasteful should not be upset if the middle-income elderly are unable to match it. Equal access to excessive technology appears to be pushing the ideal of equality a bit far.

If the bulk of the additional costly but beneficial technology represents a response to efficient demand (fueled by a growth in income, perhaps), then inequality may be more of a problem. However, we would still be left with a puzzle. If the middle class were willing to pay for beneficial but costly new technology during their working life, why should they suddenly be unwilling to do so—to such an extent as to create major apparent inequalities—when they turn 65? Why wouldn't they plan to keep up their additional insurance, especially if they are helped by a Medicare defined contribution?

A Seamless Plan

I believe that addressing this question brings us back to the rationale for Medicare in the first place. When Medicare was passed, insurance coverage, though growing, was considerably less extensive among the elderly population than among people under 65. We know two good reasons why this was so: people under 65 got a tax break for purchase of insurance—the exclusion of employment-related premiums—that the elderly did not, and the elderly were then (but are not now) poorer. Low income leads people to become uninsured in large part because the charity care option is more attractive to them than to high-income people. Because there was in 1965 a strong relationship between income levels and coverage for those over 65 suggests to me that low income (relative to fair premiums) was the primary problem. High administrative loading or adverse selection, though doubtless problems, would not have been the major causes. Adverse selection implies that the *lower* risks would go without coverage or with less-than-optimal levels of coverage, but this was not what seems to have happened.

More than thirty years later, the reasons for elderly behavior in 1965 are largely irrelevant; the question is what private insurance markets in coverage for the elderly might look like now (or even twenty years from now). If we are going to follow the defined contribution route, as we appear to be doing, de facto markets for private insurance purchasing will emerge again. I believe that improving the functioning of voluntary insurance markets is best achieved by considering methods for improvement that affect all Americans, not just (or even not especially) those over 65. In what follows, I sketch out a seamless, age-blind system of subsidies and reforms—in part based on our earlier proposals for health reform but substantially extended—that could achieve this objective (Pauly et al. 1991).

The model of a separate system of public subsidies for people over 65 is increasingly anachronistic in modern labor markets. A sizable proportion of the population retires or wishes to retire before that age, while at the same time laws are passed to forbid mandatory early retirement. What is so special about 65? Why not 55? Or 75? A better system would not have an abrupt change in subsidy status at a given age nor would it have a separate financing system. I will outline a model of a system based on extending to those over 65 the approach to universal insurance coverage that I and colleagues proposed in 1991 under the title of "Responsible National Health Insurance."

While the practical details of that scheme were complex (though much simpler than alternative NHI schemes), its design was in reality driven by two simple principles: (1) mandatory purchase of basic minimum coverage and (2) tax credits or vouchers to make compliance with the mandate affordable and easy. The required coverage for each family was the level of coverage that would assure that the family would purchase at least the levels of care socially judged to be adequate; because family circumstances vary, minimum coverage would vary as well. Such coverage would involve low cost sharing for very low-income families, but the minimum coverage whose purchase is required would fall as incomes rose. Refundable tax credits or vouchers would be tailored both to the family's income or assets *and* to the cost of the minimum coverage for the family. A key point is that the credit should rise if risk rises.

Such a model automatically accommodates the elderly: to the extent that they have low income and high risk (and therefore high fair premiums), they or the insurer they choose would be entitled to receive a larger credit than at lower risks or higher incomes. The credit could be varied in a smooth fashion, not as the all-or-nothing subsidy represented by Medicare. The credit should be lower for the better-off elderly and for those who are healthy and face low premiums. The credit would change, as a person passes from age 64 to age 65, only enough to reflect any rise in expected expense. There would be no sudden jump, no obligatory switch from one insurer to another. Indeed, it is not even obvious how great an impact age per se would have on the credit, as distinct from the effect of new chronic conditions that do accumulate with age.

Implementation Issues

The most difficult administrative problem for insurance vouchers, as for any insurance market, is how to deal with variations in risk. We have two often conflicting social goals. On the one hand, we want insurers to be eager to supply insurance to everyone, at all risk levels. On the other hand, at least some people want all persons to pay similar premiums for a given level of coverage regardless of the presence of high-risk conditions. Sometimes, such "community rating" is thought of as fair, and sometimes it is viewed as a way of insuring against the future risk of chronic conditions. Either way, it means that insurers will be forced to change premiums and sell insurance to high risks on which they will certainly lose money, a sure formula for low quality and "demarketing."

The solution to this problem in theory is simple: for all insurances (including conventional Medicare), allow the premium charged to vary with risk (risk rating) but make the credit also vary with risk (and perhaps do the same thing with minimum coverage). For instance, since risk increases with age (though in a nonlinear fashion) the credit should also increase with age. Age is easily verifiable as is gender and some other expenditure predictors. Problems arise when risk varies, given age, because of the presence of chronic conditions. It is at best extraordinarily oppressive and possibly infeasible for the government to determine whether a beneficiary really has a claimed condition or not.

What the government needs to determine, however, is not really individuals' true risks. Rather, what it needs to know is what the insurer thinks the risk is. A modest regulation would solve the problem: require insurers to post standard- and high-risk rates, and base the increment in the credit on the relative high-risk rate for those consumers who pay it. Not all of the incremental risk should be made up by the incremental credit, so that beneficiaries have an incentive to avoid being classified as high risks when they are not. The credit could either be assigned directly to the health plan or provided to the individual. In the former case, administrative costs might be lower, since there would be no need for the plan to identify to the government which of its insureds had which risk level; it would only need to tabulate the proportion of risks in each risk category. However, if we want individual beneficiaries to be able to shop effectively, we will have to tell them what size credit to expect.

Such an integration of subsidization for insurance at all ages would actually have little or no effect on current tax rates because the amount of the current tax subsidy for purchase of insurance by employed people under age 65—directed toward higher-income people who buy lavish coverage—is adequate to provide a generous subsidy to low-income people (depending, of course, on the politically chosen level of minimum coverage and maximum subsidy).

How would such a system fare over time? For one thing, it would make the level of technological change, at all ages, a matter of social choice: what improvements in new technology would be included in the minimum package and what level of subsidy and/or coverage they would receive would have to be considered in setting the credit and minimum coverage. The political choice would be as rational as such choices can be for the under-65 population, since in large part the beneficiaries would pay the cost immediately. The more heavily subsidized coverage for over 65s would continue to be less directly constrained, but now the link with beneficiary-financed coverage would serve to constrain and equalize as well.

People would be motivated to budget at all ages for the portion of the premiums of the required coverage they would have to pay, with the well-off paying almost all of the premium and a gradual increase in subsidy as income falls. Demographic change would mean an increase in the proportion of higher-risk people for whom the credit would presumably be more generous. If increasingly costly technology is chosen, it would only be because taxpayers can "afford it"—and they would save privately to even out net consumption. In short, the separate problem of paying for Medicare would disappear, to be replaced by the more general problem of choosing and then financing subsidies in a society in which there are moderate increases in the proportion of the population needing a subsidy—hopefully matched with a rate of real growth in total income sufficient to finance those subsidies and improvements in quality at higher cost. Tautologically but truly, the subsidies would be chosen only because they could be financed; there would be no prospect of a phony bankruptcy or sudden jumps in taxes caused by an ersatz trust fund.

The intergenerational issue would, however, still remain: taxpayers who grew up paying a fairly small tax could, as they age in larger proportions and if they fail to save, impose a heavier burden on their less numerous children. In principle, this would be incorporated by projecting smaller credits and lower coverage across the board in the future (not just for the elderly); the smaller credits relative to the premium should trigger increased voluntary saving (and investment in private market instruments) for people who want to be able to pay higher future private premiums. The problem of financing for the elderly becomes the broader problem of lifetime saving and consumption planning in a world in which obligatory payments (taxes and premiums) are expected to rise.

I do not claim that this scheme makes the Medicare/demographic bogeyman go away. It does not, although it blends one scare with some others and with greater certainty about what a future with mixed blessings will bring. Taxing based on wealth as well as income may help to smooth year-to-year fluctuations in taxes somewhat. In contrast to a mandatory savings program, such as that proposed by Gramm, Rettenmaier, and Saving (1998), this scheme does not force down consumption during a middle-income person's working lifetime to avoid making transfers to that person if they choose to have a lower income upon retirement. Use of a consumption tax would help even more and might solve the problem. To generate high transfers to myself when I retire, I would have to consume more heavily in my youth and pass my retirement consuming the memories of past consumption—not an especially attractive prospect to many people, I suspect. We could wait to see whether mandatory savings is required to keep retiree income up enough so that they can pay for their own coverage.

Subsidies and Savings: A Lifetime Perspective

Suppose then a subsidy program exists that will make higher payments to people with lower income and higher risk, regardless of age. Agents know that their risk will rise with age. Income in any time period depends on work and investment income, and investment income in turn depends on prior saving. How will the subsidy affect a person's lifetime planning?

Absent the subsidy, the income planned for the older-age period would have to be enough to cover all consumption items during that period, both medical and nonmedical. Planned and desired medical consumption rises with age; we assume that optimal values of other consumption are independent of age. These considerations imply that total income must rise with age; saving will have to occur early in life to provide the resources for medical care.

Now suppose a credit is offered that effectively increases with age and declines with income or consumption. The credit does not discourage saving if the credit varies proportionately with consumption, if the desired level of health spending exceeds the credit in every period, and if the credit is a linear function of consumption. This is because the credit depends only on lifetime income and lifetime medical risk. Consuming more when young so as to have lower income (be more needy) when old is not advantageous, since lower credits when young offset higher credits when old.

However, things change if credits are not (inversely) proportional to consumption. Then planning a few very needy periods may increase the total lifetime flow of credits. This is much easier to do if credits depend on income rather than on consumption, since it is less painful to stop income than to stop consumption. If credits are a function of consumption, the key issue is the substitutability of consumption in one period for that in others. The net effect is like a progressive tax on consumption—bothersome but not obviously lethal.

The fact that rising wealth or income upon retirement would, under an income-conditioned program, reduce social insurance benefits would be expected to cause a disincentive to earn money income and to save. Feldstein (1987) cautions against means-tested Social Security on this score, although obviously the ultimate question is empirical: Would a pattern of net benefits that decreased with income or wealth upon retirement discourage work effort during one's productive years by more than a lower average tax rate would encourage it? Neumark and Powers (1997) offer evidence that (for Social Security) work effort is discouraged given some level of payroll taxes. They do not provide quantitative estimates of the magnitude or of the overall effect.

However, Medicare differs from Social Security in two different ways. First, at present Social Security benefits increase with earnings (though not proportionately) up to a point, while the nominal value of Medicare benefits is independent of income. This means that switching to a means-tested benefit pattern is a larger change in net benefits related to income for Social Security than for Medicare. Second, there is reason to believe that Medicare coverage for higher-income beneficiaries presently is inefficiently large (so there is an efficiency gain from cutting benefits back), whereas there is no reason to believe that Social Security pensions for higher-wage workers are excessive.

All of this does, however, assume rationality. What about the person who earns a decent income and consumes well when working but who foolishly does not save for retirement? This person will, because of low retirement income and wealth, trigger a larger credit than if he or she has been forced to save. But is forcing the person to save for Medicare a good solution? We are back to the paternalism argument, but in this case information—how miserable you can be if you do not save and live too long—could be an alternative stimulus. Perhaps people will respond to that information.

It would seem that offering income-related credits, even if they are generous enough to cause the average person at any income level to buy at least minimum coverage, may still necessitate mandatory purchase to get universal coverage. Perhaps not necessarily; Medicare Part B is not mandated but participation is still virtually universal—but the subsidy is 75 percent.

What if people foolishly choose not to even out their lifetime consumption and income, and so are low-income retirees? The paternalistic spirit behind Social Security and Medicare Part A is that they should nevertheless be required to pay when they are young to have more income and benefits when they are old; the current controversy (on both subjects) is how the proceeds of those compulsory payments (taxes) should be invested. Just as there is a paternalistic basis for requiring provisions of higher levels of income in general after retirement (Social Security), there might be a similar basis (whatever it is) for requiring an earmarked fund for health insurance.

Comparison with the Current System

The system of income-conditioned coverage and credits I have proposed is in some ways similar to the current system and in other ways very different. The main similarity is that the great majority of elders will be required to obtain health insurance with a prespecified level of coverage, and they will receive partial government subsidies for doing so (just as in today's Medicare) but also be required to pay some of the premium for this insurance themselves (just as in today's Medicare). They will have the same kind of choices of suppliers for this insurance as they have in today's Medicare (after the Balanced Budget Act [BBA]): they may choose indemnity insurance supplied by HCFA; managed care plans; or private insurers offering indemnity, managed indemnity, or provider-sponsored coverage. All of the still troublesome issues about risk-adjusting the government contribution and informing beneficiaries will apply to my scheme as well.

There is, however, an important difference: The scope of the mandated coverage I propose will not have just two steps as it does now

(Medicaid plus Medicare for the poor; Medicare for everyone else); instead, it will have many steps and include truly catastrophic coverage for the high-income normal risks. Higher-wealth people are permitted to buy catastrophic coverage only, instead of getting the same generous Medicare policy that lower-income people are offered. (The MSA experiment does offer catastrophic coverage to a limited number of beneficiaries now, but it does not condition eligibility on income as my proposal would do.) As a practical step, or as an interim step, it might be better to design several discrete versions of catastrophic plans and assign income-risk categories to each, rather than construct the more complex continuous variation. Moreover, although this is a matter ultimately of social judgment, it may be that the beneficiary's share of the premium for the mandated coverage I propose will be greater at higher-income levels than it is now (but, on the other hand, the total premium will be lower).

In this scheme, as in any scheme that tries to use markets to supply insurance, the most devilish detail is how to treat variation in risk. High risks get different treatment in this scheme. They are required to buy more coverage than otherwise similar people of lower risk, but they receive larger subsidies to help them do so. Serious design questions include how to measure risk; what, if anything, to do about supplemental insurance people of different risk levels may buy; and what aspects of risk to adjust for.

The answers to all of these design questions are both debatable and distracting. Here are some preliminary answers. First, perfect risk adjustment is neither required nor expected; adjustment based on systems now in place seem to do a reasonable job of getting government payments close to "constant-quality" cost at each risk level, and small errors need only result in small quality or beneficiary premium variations. That is, if we oversubsidize a little for some person, the only result will be that his or her mandated coverage will be a little cheaper or a little better than average—as long as insurance markets are as competitive as we expect them to be. Second, high risks would be required to buy higher levels of coverage, given income, than lower risks, but they would not be subsidized to buy unlimited levels of coverage; they would be permitted to buy supplementary coverage if they wished, but there would be no need to risk-adjust the premiums for that coverage since, by definition, it covers care of little social concern. Finally, it would seem sensible to adjust the credit for risks related to health but not those related to tastes. If, for example, whites tend to use more care, given insurance coverage and everything else, than do nonwhites, that would not entitle whites to larger credits, even though insurers might tend to charge higher premiums for the mandated coverage in market areas where whites predominate. Actually making the right discrimination in geographic adjustments will be tricky but not impossible. An even more perplexing case is associated with the fact that the market premium for a policy chosen by higher-income people will tend to be higher than the premium would be for such a policy if it had been chosen by lower-income people. Should the credit then be increased for the higher-income people? My preliminary answer to such questions is that the risk adjustments should probably be generated by the effect of a set of "legitimate" risk characteristics (diabetes is allowed as a risk adjuster; a history of hypochondria or a demonstrated taste for expensive doctors, is not) applied to the health care expenses of the entire elderly population under various insurance policies. This is a large actuarial task but is not an insurmountable one—and will, in any case, have to be addressed after the BBA under current legislation.

My proposal generally expands the choices offered to most (though not all) Americans. Except for the very rich, elders will still be required to obtain some insurance; they cannot choose to be uninsured. They may select the mandated insurance from the same types of options as they currently can. They may also choose (or not choose) to buy supplemental coverage; that market is currently regulated fairly heavily, for some good reasons, but some relaxation might be possible. I would propose that those who buy supplemental coverage be allowed to be charged a higher premium by the supplier of their mandated coverage, to reflect the expected heavier use of that coverage; in this sense, the artificial subsidy to supplemental coverage would be stopped. In practical terms, it may be that people will be required to buy their supplemental coverage from the same insurer as they use for their mandated coverage in order to enforce such policies. Higher-income people will have the opportunity to choose insurance plans with less lavish coverage than Medicare currently provides. This option is currently limited to those who select MSAs; my proposals would extend this privilege (without the inequitable payroll tax–financed MSA deposits to the accounts of high-income persons) to many more beneficiaries. However, in contrast to the MSA experiment, it would forbid lower-income or higher-risk beneficiaries from choosing catastrophic coverage in order to save money, since the potential for underuse of care by those persons should be minimized.

Limiting mandated coverage to adequate coverage and subsidizing it appropriately will lead people to choose to consume adequate amounts of medical services, and thus satisfy what was assumed to be the main social objective of the Medicare program. It will, however, allow much more of the insurance purchasing of middle- and upper-income elders to be made outside the social insurance framework, in a private market for supplemental coverage. There are reasons to expect that if this market is left unregulated and unsubsidized, some people will have problems. Administrative costs for individually marketed and voluntarily purchased private insurance are likely to be high, and market premiums may vary with risk. These characteristics are exactly the supposed defects in the Medigap market that federal regulations are designed to limit; in the proposed new scheme, because the scope of supplemental insurance is potentially larger (though not necessarily so), more insurance may be obtained in a private market that, even with regulation, is thought by many to function less well than Medicare. People underusing care will not be a problem, but there could be a problem of people paying too much (by a number of different definitions) for the insurance covering care that is not a matter of high social concern.

Doesn't this still leave a malfunctioning market that would not have to exist if only everyone got almost all of their insurance from the government system, as at present? Continuing the current system is not an option. One's answer to this question turns on judgments about how well the government would manage a severely constrained Medicare system and how well one expects markets to perform. Medicare is not perfectly administered, and may be even less well administered when it has to accommodate the options of Medicare+Choice, but the private market surely is not perfect either. Current knowledge does not allow us to answer the question of which is (second) best. However, the gain from saving mandated coverage seems to me to be greater than the risk that there will be some moderate additional inefficiency in the market for supplemental coverage. Others may see the odds differently.

Conclusion

I have argued for the desirability of income-related subsidies and income-related coverage for Medicare beneficiaries. Implementation of such a change immediately, though justified as a way of "saving the trust fund," is sure to be controversial and revolutionary. This argues for a gradual phase-in of new arrangements but announcement of the phase-in schedule now.

The Medicare financing discussion throws into sharp focus two aspects of social policy that are themselves confused. First, what do we mean by adequate care that we are willing to pay for? Second, what values do we place on beneficial but costly new technology? Treating these questions separately for the elderly has the advantage of limited scope but the disadvantage of irrationality. It would be best to consider health reform (and re-reform) as all of a piece.

Notes

1. Ideally, the transformation from tax to subsidy should be a smooth and continuous function of age, not abrupt as it currently is for Medicare (but not Social Security). More on this below.

2. The technical arrangement is as follows: If people are buying coverage at the margin with their own money, the value of an additional unit of coverage is worth its full cost. But then the marginal value to the community must be zero, so no subsidy is needed.

References

Board of Trustees, Federal Hospital Insurance Trust Fund. 1997. *The 1997 Annual Report of the Board of Trustees of the Federal Hospital Insurance Trust Fund* (24 April).

Feldstein, M. S. 1987. "Should Social Security Benefits Be Means Tested?" *Journal of Political Economy* 95 (3): 468–84.

Feldstein, P. 1988. *Health Care Economics,* 3rd edition. Albany: Delmar Publishers.

Gramm, W. P., A. J. Rettenmaier, and T. R. Saving. 1998. "Medicare Policy for Future Generations—A Search for a Permanent Solution." *New England Journal of Medicine* 338 (18, 30 April): 1,307–10.

Hadley, J. 1982. *More Medical Care, Better Health?: An Economic Analysis of Mortality Rates*. Washington, D.C.: Urban Institute Press.

McClellan, M., and J. Skinner. 1997. "The Incidence of Medicare." NBER Working Paper 6013, April.

Neumark, D., and E. Powers. 1997. "Means Testing Social Security." *PRC WP* 17–24. Philadelphia: Pension Research Council.

Newhouse, J. et al. 1993. *Free for All: Lessons from the RAND Health Insurance Experiment?* Cambridge: Harvard University Press.

Pauly, M. V. 1971. *Medical Care at Public Expense*. New York: Praeger Publishers, Inc.

———. 1995. "When Does Curbing Health Costs Really Help the Economy?" *Health Affairs* 14 (2): 68–82.

———. 1996. "Will Medicare Reforms Increase Managed Care Enrollment?" *Health Affairs* 15 (3): 182–91.

Pauly, M. V., P. Danzon, P. Feldstein, and J. Hoff. 1991. "A Plan for 'Responsible National Health Insurance.'" *Health Affairs* 10 (1): 5–25.

Peden, E. A., and M. S. Freeland. 1995. "A Historical Analysis of Medical Spending Growth." *Health Affairs* 14 (2): 235–47.

Phelps, C. E. 1997. *Health Economics,* 2nd ed. New York: Addison-Wesley.

Reischauer, R. D. 1997a. "Midnight Follies." *Washington Post* (22 June), p. C7.

———. 1997b. "Medicare, Beyond 2002: Preparing for the Baby Boomers." *New York Times* (22 June), sec. 3, p. 24.

Chapter Four

Comment: The Limits of Economic Incentives

Marilyn Moon

At a conference devoted to examining the economics of Medicare, it is dangerous to suggest that there are limitations to what markets and market incentives can accomplish. But that is the issue I want to stress in my remarks. I do not doubt the strength of market forces and the enormous possibilities for generating efficient solutions to many problems. But in health care, efficiency is not as likely to be a goal prized by consumers in the same way as for other products. Other factors need to be brought into the equation as well. A broader policy analysis of what new factors need to be brought to bear and what will work can help ground the pure economics in the art of the practical.

The three papers I discuss here illustrate issues surrounding the use of economic incentives to justify public policy changes. Mark V. Pauly offers the traditional neoclassical economic approach in his chapter about how generous Medicare should be for higher-income beneficiaries. As a consequence, I particularly focus on some of the issues left out of Pauly's analysis. Henry J. Aaron and Victor R. Fuchs, on the other hand, also question whether we should look only at incentives, competition, and other traditional economic principles in seeking solutions to Medicare's financing problems.

From my prospective, several key questions must be added to any pure economic analysis:

- How should we trade off competing desires to improve incentives when there are actually multiple goals and multiple instruments for achieving those goals?
- How do we establish priorities across various goals?

Marilyn Moon is a senior fellow at the Urban Institute in Washington, D.C.

- How do we balance the goals of efficiency with other legitimate concerns that are usually ignored in standard economic theory, including the distribution of resources and desires to share such resources in various ways?

Numerous studies of Medicare beneficiaries and consumers in general suggest that consumption of health care exceeds the optimal or most efficient amount. Some of this reflects individual behaviors in the face of subsidized prices because of insurance and third-party payers. Some reflects excess use that may be a proxy for quality; consumers who have poor information may opt for too much rather than too little care. Some reflects the incentives that providers face in a fee-for-service world to maximize the number of services offered. Some reflects fraudulent activities on the part of suppliers to inappropriately increase the use of services.

What then do economists offer to address the issue of overuse? Consider first the issue of the benefit package and Medicare. Both Aaron and Pauly cite the inefficiency of a two-part system of Medicare and private supplemental policies (both individually purchased Medigap policies and employer-subsidized retiree benefits). Medicare's cost sharing is often recognized as being too high and out of sync with other insurance policies. But the response has been to supplement Medicare in ways that eliminate nearly all cost sharing, thus encouraging the consumption of too much care. And much of the cost of any excess use of care is borne by the Medicare program rather than by the supplemental policies encouraging such activity.

Applied Neoclassical Economics

Pauly's solution is to focus on the upper end of the income scale and reduce substantially the subsidy that Medicare provides to such persons. Although such proposals are often made on equity grounds, Pauly justifies his proposal on efficiency grounds and in fact stresses that criterion over and above issues of redistribution. Pauly correctly points out that higher-income persons are more likely to have supplemental policies and ones that are more generous than those available to lower-income persons. Employer-subsidized plans are more often found among this income group. The usual approach to such an analysis is to propose taxing supplemental policies or assessing taxes directly on high-income individuals. Instead, however, Pauly argues that the only feasible way to improve efficiency is to move Medicare to a defined contribution system of vouchers in which the voucher amount declines with income. Thus, he would totally change the Medicare program to achieve greater efficiency for this one portion of the Medicare population.

What Pauly discounts, however, is how important this goal is relative to the overarching principles that justify the very popular current structure of the Medicare program. That is, the universal nature of the program was and is no accident. Many of its supporters feel adamant about the support that such universality achieves for this social insurance program. A comprehensive discussion of such a massive change in the program needs to be put in a much broader context. Other reasons for moving to a voucher system would have to be explored and justified before taking such a proposal seriously.

Further, vouchers would shift a universal program with low administrative costs into an individual insurance market with all of the well-noted inefficiencies of marketing costs, high overhead, and administrative expenses. Just on *efficiency* grounds, such a proposal may be unwise.

Who should be subject to reduced subsidies? Who gets defined as "less worthy" of protection? In theory, one of the difficulties with penalizing higher-income individuals is the conflict that arises in terms of offering incentives for older Americans to save for their retirement. If higher incomes in retirement mean that they will face lower Medicare protections, rational individuals may decline to postpone consumption in earlier years if they feel that such sacrifices will not be rewarded in the future. Concern about the national savings rate is certainly a conflicting goal in this context. And as Medicare becomes a larger and larger program relative to the size of income of the elderly, this conflict is heightened.

On the practical side, when people discuss some type of income or means testing, they quickly discover that Medicare saves little; there simply are not enough high-income seniors to generate massive savings (Moon 1996). This calls into question whether the goal of reducing subsidies for those with high incomes justifies such massive changes in the Medicare program. Pauly's approach is to begin to phase out the subsidies for persons with incomes above 300 percent of the official poverty level. In 1998 that would be less than $25,000 for a single person and about $32,000 for a couple. This would capture a larger share of the senior population, but by most definitions such individuals would not be considered wealthy—particularly since individuals in that income range would be faced with very high health spending burdens.

Beyond Economics

Aaron's chapter in many ways takes off where Pauly's ends, exploring how much choice among health plans to offer beneficiaries. Aaron also takes a very different approach to the issue of improving the efficiency of the Medicare program. He would expand and modify the basic benefit package so as to eliminate the need for the inefficient supplemental insurance policies. This constitutes an expansion and strengthening of the Medicare program rather than turning immediately to a private sector, laissez-faire approach. In fact, Aaron challenges the notion that choice is necessarily a good thing for the Medicare program, particularly in its broadest form. His criticism of those who assert that unlimited choice is inherently a better approach to organizing health care without providing solid evidence for that claim is certainly consistent with my own skepticism about the market for health care.

Aaron marshals a great deal of support through examples and specific suggestions for other factors that need to be brought to bear to assess whether choice itself is a means for generating a more efficient and improved Medicare program. He addresses the practical problems that choice creates in the current system from our inability to adjust payments for health status and for the subsequent varying expenditure needs of Medicare beneficiaries. This inability leads to overpayment of private plans and perverse incentives to attract healthy enrollees.

But much of Aaron's analysis demands that we expand beyond basic economic theory to entertain the possibilities of other goals and other criteria for judging policy. In particular, I am struck by his defense of paternalism—in this case, another way of expressing that what is good for some individuals may not be good for society as a whole. Economic theory is cognizant of market failures and externalities, but too often enthusiasm for the elegance of the basic theory causes economists to overlook these messy caveats.

Nonetheless, rather than reject a market approach, Aaron seeks to offer modifications that could mitigate its negative effects and harness the savings and efficiencies that could follow. This is one of his reasons for stressing a uniform and expanded benefit package. I, too, have become convinced that this is a major issue; it is difficult to expect markets to deal with differences in benefit packages. Consider, for example, prescription drugs. This benefit, now excluded from the basic Medicare package, is increasingly viewed as essential to effective health care delivery. But it is also a magnet for riskier patients when offered either by private supplemental plans (Medigap) or by the managed care plans that now cover the full range of Medicare benefits and often offer additional benefits to attract enrollees. Left to itself, over time, the likely market response will be to eliminate or severely limit coverage of drugs by both types of plans.

The key unanswered question for Aaron is whether his modifications on choice will truly be enough to result in a well-functioning market in an expanded choice environment. His arguments about the pitfalls are compelling. Will controls on the benefit package and improvements in payments to those plans by the federal government be sufficient to overcome the substantial problems he foresees? It is extremely unlikely that future reforms of Medicare will fully undo choice, so Aaron's approach to placing reasonable limits on it seems to be the appropriate direction, but I suspect we may need even more vigilance than he anticipates.

A Holistic Approach

The first chapter, by Victor Fuchs, takes a more holistic view of the problem, casting it more in the light of what the elderly themselves and we as a society wish to—and are able to—afford. Fuchs's tables remind us that it is difficult to continue on the path of our recent history of "relentless increase in consumption of health care by older Americans." But I would go further and suggest that it is not just the elderly who are avid consumers of health care, but rather most Americans (Altman and Wallack 1996). As a society, we applaud the development of new treatments and products and clamor to use them whenever possible. Health care spending growth is found throughout the health care system and not just in Medicare or for seniors. The dilemma of whether we will continue to expand our resources to consume a greater and greater share of GDP in the form of health care is an extremely important question, but one that must be played out well beyond the bounds of the Medicare program. It is in this area that Fuchs stresses the need for careful monitoring of economic incentives.

Fuchs is less prescriptive regarding other solutions than are Pauly and Aaron. The two areas he stresses needing the greatest attention are encouragement of more years of work by individuals who on average are living longer and more savings in order to support the types of health care consumption we seem to desire. Here again is an area where economic incentives could be used, and Fuchs advocates reducing some of the high marginal tax rates now facing older workers. This seems to be in contrast to others who are increasingly pushing for a compulsory approach through an increase in the age of eligibility for the program, thus requiring individuals to find insurance elsewhere before age 67 or 70. Fuchs leaves open the ultimate questions of how we as a society decide to share resources across generations, but his chapter certainly provides provocative findings that various combatants on all sides will be able to use in the upcoming debate. The most compelling finding from my perspective is the likely limit on what burdens we can expect the elderly themselves to bear.

Economics and Health Care

Health care is not like many other goods or services; consumers do not always want to use care just to the point where marginal revenues are equal to marginal costs. In fact, redundancies are often valued for their option value in health care. That is, we wish to have too many hospital beds for those rare times when catastrophic events would otherwise overwhelm our medical system. At any one point in time, waiting your turn is not an acceptable solution. Moreover, many consumers would like to have more tests than may be optimal from a pure efficiency standpoint. Some of this particular inefficiency likely stems from the existence of third-party payers, who shield consumers from the full costs of their care. But even when the consumer is paying the full cost, desires to overconsume health care services will likely continue. Information and certainty about outcomes are particularly poor in health care and the consequences of underservice are potentially devastating. Such overuse is a critical proxy for quality; and until better measures and information about quality and effectiveness are available, this will be a safety valve that consumers demand. Thus, I believe that as a society we are not only willing but anxious to forgo some of the efficiencies that a market brings.

We ignore these desires at our peril in designing new policy approaches. Many consumers will be skeptical of solutions offered for the express purpose of improving efficiency, perhaps helping to explain some of the current dissatisfaction with managed care. Medical savings accounts, reducing subsidies for high-income Medicare beneficiaries, and more choice among plans, for example, all suffer as proposals for reform from the perspective that they are often promoted as good economics, without taking into account the fact that it is not just efficiency that people want in their health care system.

Further, the institutional and other constraints facing the delivery of health care also mitigate against a total free market approach to solving some of the problems facing Medicare in the future. Providing health care coverage for older and disabled persons is well accepted as a role for government. The private sector has never served these populations well; the ability to divide the risk pool in serving sicker populations is a much more attractive way for insurers to make money than to find more efficient ways to deliver care. The resulting market failure poses formidable barriers for generating alternative approaches to serving this population, and any new proposal ought to be judged against that standard. Practical considerations often cast great doubt on approaches that, in theory, sound desirable.

Finally, the issue of intergenerational concerns and the aging of the population certainly are creating challenges for the Medicare program. But these are largely distributional questions of who should pay that pure economic analysis is also poorly equipped to handle. While one set of solutions for Medicare's future financing problems is surely to seek to more efficiently deliver care, the fact is that even if we slow the growth in the costs of care substantially, new products and treatments will be desired by consumers. Further, a greater number of elderly persons in the future suggests that we will and should devote a greater share of national income to health care for the elderly. This suggests that Medicare should not be condemned just because it is large and growing; rather, we need to find ways to meet the financing challenges ahead.

Economic analysis is a crucial component of the policy debate that should take place around Medicare. But it is not and cannot be sufficient to address all the issues important for designing policies for the twenty-first century. At a minimum, intergenerational distributional issues, institutional factors, and desires by consumers for some inefficiencies ought to be given attention as well.

References

Altman, Stuart, and Stanley Wallack. 1996. "Health Care Spending: Can the United States Control It?" In *Strategic Choices for a Changing Health Care System*, edited by Stuart Altman and Uwe Reinhardt. *The Baxter Health Policy Review,* vol. II. Chicago: Health Administration Press.

Moon, Marilyn. 1996. Medicare Now and in the Future, 2nd edition. Washington, D.C.: The Urban Institute Press.

Chapter Five

Does Ownership Affect the Cost of Medicare?

Frank A. Sloan
Donald H. Taylor Jr.

I. Introduction

Unlike most other sectors in which firms are organized as for-profit enterprises, U.S. hospitals are heterogeneous in their ownership and sponsorship. In terms of ownership, the majority of hospitals, 60 percent, are organized as private nonprofit organizations, with public hospitals, 28 percent, being second most frequent. For-profit hospitals are third with a market share of 12 percent. Shares by ownership have been remarkably stable over the second half of this century (American Hospital Association 1998).

Ownership is a potentially important determinant of hospital behavior for these reasons. In a for-profit enterprise, the residual claimants are the shareholders. Thus, if the organization is either inefficient or cross-subsidizes an unprofitable activity, profits accruing to the claimant are correspondingly reduced on a dollar-to-dollar basis. By contrast, charters of private nonprofit organizations forbid private

Frank A. Sloan is the J. Alexander McMahon Professor of Health Policy and Management, professor of economics, and director of the Center for Health Policy, Law and Management at Duke University.

Donald H. Taylor Jr. is an assistant research professor of public policy studies at Duke University and a member of the Center for Health Policy, Law and Management, Duke University.

Research for this study was supported in part by a grant from the National Institute on Aging to Duke University. We thank Shin-Yi Chou for capable research assistance.

inurement. Thus, the managers generally do not benefit personally from improved efficiency or reductions in cross subsidies.[1] Although the community is legally the owner, an operational definition of community is often lacking (Sloan, Taylor, and Conover 1997). Further, groups representing the collective interest of community members may not be sufficiently well organized to adequately represent the interests of its constituents. Since a dollar's increase in waste or in a cross subsidy does not accrue as a loss to a well-defined or organized group of constituents, the managers may "buy" extra waste or units of various cross-subsidized activities. At least some of the latter is often viewed as socially desirable and is often cited as an explanation of the dominance of the private nonprofit form in the hospital sector.[2] Another factor possibly contributing to the dominance of the nonprofit form relates to competitive advantages. Unlike their for-profit counterparts, private nonprofit organizations do not pay property or corporate income taxes and are eligible for private donations. They have some advantages in their ability to issue tax-exempt debt as well. Relative to for-profits, they are disadvantaged in their inability to issue equity (Institute of Medicine 1986).

Diffuse constituency also applies to public hospitals, but at least for such organizations there is political accountability. Public hospitals are also tax exempt and are more likely to receive public subsidies and less likely to receive private donations than are private nonprofit hospitals.

Important among activities subsidized by hospitals are jointly produced teaching and unsponsored research. Although the exact amounts are not known, these activities presumably require cross subsidies in part because students are inexperienced clinicians and require supervision. Further, as part of the learning process, students order various procedures that would not be ordered by more experienced physicians. Care provided at teaching hospitals is also said to be more costly because (1) they treat cases that are more complex to diagnose and treat and (2) their quality of care may be higher (Lave 1985; Physician Payment Review Commission 1997, 382–88; Welch 1987). Such activity may be measured in various ways. In this chapter, we follow Medicare's convention and define the amount of this activity in terms of the ratio of full-time equivalent interns and residents to beds.

Medicare has traditionally developed specific payment policies dependent on hospital ownership and teaching status. Historically, Medicare paid for-profit hospitals an explicit return on equity. This subsidy is no longer paid. Until 1992, depreciation, interest, rent, and certain property-related expenses for insurance and taxes were paid by Medicare on a retrospective cost basis. To the extent that for-profit hospitals borrowed at higher interest rates and/or received payments for added taxes they paid, this would have been reflected in a higher Medicare payment. Under the system that replaced retrospective payment for capital, fixed capital payments per case were slightly higher for for-profit than for nonprofit hospitals. Public hospitals, especially those in rural areas, were paid much less.[3] Teaching hospitals are paid by Medicare on a retrospective cost basis for direct medical education (DME) cost—salaries and benefits to residents and faculty, classroom costs, and associated overhead—and according to a formula for indirect medical education (IME) cost, the latter based on the hospital's ratio of interns and residents to beds.[4] There is some debate about whether IME represents payment for an added cost of patient care because of, among other reasons, a more complex case mix not accounted for by diagnosis-related groups (DRGs). Alternatively, IME may be payment for something else, such as a higher-quality level or inefficiencies attributable to teaching not covered from other sources.[5]

Another Medicare subsidy is for hospitals that provide a disproportionate share of care (DSH) to Medicare and Medicaid patients. The DSH adjustment is intended to provide extra compensation to hospitals that serve a disproportionate share of low-income patients. To the extent that some types of hospitals provide more of such care than others, these payments may differ systematically by ownership and location (Prospective Payment Assessment Commission 1997, 69–72).

Although the U.S. hospital industry has been the object of much study, considerable controversy remains about the relative performance of hospitals, both in terms of cost and quality, especially along dimensions of ownership and teaching status. In practical terms, the controversy has reached the general public's attention in recent years because of allegations of fraud on the part of Columbia/HCA, the largest for-profit hospital company, and the increased pace of hospital ownership conversions that has affected many communities throughout the United States.[6]

This chapter uses panel data on Medicare beneficiaries to investigate these issues. First, how does ownership and teaching status of the hospital at which a beneficiary is hospitalized affect Medicare payments, holding other factors constant? By payments, we include the index (first) hospitalization and other payments made for care rendered during the first six months following the date of the index admission. Where differences are observed, we investigate sources of such differences. Although Medicare pays a fixed price per case, there are nevertheless ways that payment flows can be influenced. The same incentive that may lead profit-seeking hospitals to be efficient may lead such hospitals to influence cash flows from programs such as Medicare. This might be accomplished by upcoding diagnoses or by referral patterns during and following the index admission. The rapid growth in post-acute care following implementation of the Medicare Prospective Payment System (PPS) is probably in part a response to financial incentives that PPS provides to unbundle hospital services (Prospective Payment Assessment Commission 1997). The increase in rehabilitative services provided to Medicare beneficiaries since PPS was implemented is a case in point (Welch et al. 1996; Kramer et al. 1997; Chan et al. 1997). The strength of the data used in this study is in allowing us to disentangle the various avenues by which payments may be increased.

Second, do outcomes differ by hospital ownership and teaching status? Outcomes are measured in terms of mortality, rehospitalization, probability of living in the community rather than in a nursing home, and various measures of functional status measured in the months and up to a few years following the index admission. We limit our analysis to patients over age 65, all enrolled in Medicare, who were hospitalized following four types of adverse health events involving a broken hip, a stroke, coronary heart disease including heart attacks, and congestive heart failure. We ask if Medicare paid more in the six months following the adverse event if the patient was first admitted to a for-profit facility.

Section II describes our data. In section III, we discuss the specification of the equations used to measure the effects of ownership and teaching status on performance. Section IV presents empirical results. And in section V, we discuss the implications of our findings for an understanding of the role of ownership in hospital payment and for Medicare policy in particular.

II. Data

The study sample was drawn from the National Long-Term Care Survey (NLTCS), which is a panel study fielded in 1982, 1984, 1989, and 1994. Overall, 35,800 Medicare beneficiaries were included in the database for at least some time. NLTCS randomly drew its sample from Medicare enrollment records for persons 65 years of age and older. A screener interview was administered to those selected. Based on responses to the screener, full interviews were conducted with persons who reported having at least one chronic limitation in activities of daily living (ADLs) or in instrumental activities of daily living (IADLs). The ADLs were using help for eating, getting in or out of bed, moving around inside, dressing, bathing, and using the toilet (maximum of six). The IADLs were using help for doing housework, preparing meals, shopping for groceries, managing their money, moving independently outside, and taking medicine (maximum of six) (Katz and Akpo 1976).[7] Given the high rate of mortality in this population, it was essential to replace decedents with new (to the sample) beneficiaries. This was done in successive waves; in 1989, 4,900 new persons who had "aged-in" to the sample selection criteria were screened, as were 4,500 persons in 1994 (National Institute on Aging 1998). Respondents lived in the community or elsewhere, most notably in nursing homes. The NLTCS collected detailed information on functional and cognitive status; health conditions; demographic characteristics of the family, including potential caregivers; years of schooling completed; race/ethnicity; and income, including sources of income, and wealth.

The NLTCS was merged with data from other sources. First, data on all Medicare claims, inpatient, outpatient, Part B physician, home health, skilled nursing facility, and hospice from 1982 through 1995 were merged with all individuals screened by NLTCS in any year (Manton and Stallard 1991; Manton et al. 1995). Each claim included information on diagnoses, amounts billed and paid by Medicare, measures of quantity and dates of service, and some demographic characteristics. Using hospital identifiers on the claim, we could identify the hospitals, which in turn allowed us to assign ownership codes using data from the American Hospital Association (AHA). Also using AHA data, we assigned values of the resident-to-bed ratio by hospital and year as a measure of the intensity of teaching activity at the hospital. Dates of deaths for all NLTCS respondents are contained on the NLTCS analytical file and have been verified by using Medicare enrollment records, the National Death Index, and state vital records systems for all respondents to the NLTCS.

For purposes of this analysis, we selected persons who were admitted to hospitals with primary diagnoses of hip fracture, stroke, coronary heart disease, or congestive heart failure[8] for stays of 91 days or less; individuals dying on the date of index admission were included if they were admitted. We selected the first admission for these conditions that occurred starting in 1984. Since Medicare claims data starting in 1982 were available and the NLTCS asked about conditions during the preceding year, we had a minimum of a three-year look-back period for ascertaining "first" admissions for a particular condition. The 1982 wave of NLTCS was only used for purposes of selecting the sample. A purpose for limiting the empirical analysis to first admissions for the tracer conditions was to reduce omitted heterogeneity. For example, persons may select a hospital for a hard-to-treat condition after care at other hospitals failed to yield desired results.

For measuring rehospitalization, there had to be at least three days between a discharge and a subsequent admission. This criterion was selected because patients were sometimes shown by Medicare claims data as discharged and readmitted to the same hospital on the same day; these cases likely represented transfers between units within the same hospital or transfers to other types of facilities to continue care (such as a rehabilitation hospital).

We screened hospitalizations for the study conditions to exclude cases with missing Medicare payment data or cases with less than $10 payment for an index admission. Cases were also excluded from our sample if they could not be merged to a prior NLTCS full interview or screener interview; such data were necessary for pre-index hospitalization measures of health and functional status (for example, ADLs, cognition, lived-in community). This initial selection process yielded a total of 3,191 observations, including 795 for hip fracture, 790 for stroke, 1,001 for coronary heart disease, and 605 for congestive heart failure. Some beneficiaries were admitted to hospitals for more than one of these primary diagnoses. In such cases, we took the first study event that occurred. Five hundred seventeen index admissions for study conditions were dropped from the analysis because they represented individuals who had previously had an index admission for another study condition. This case selection process resulted in a pooled analysis sample of 2,674 who were admitted to 1,378 different hospitals throughout the United States. Once a case was selected, it was followed through the end of 1995 or death, whichever occurred first. The full pooled sample was used to analyze Medicare payments, survival, and rehospitalization. Numbers of observations for analysis of the probability of remaining a community resident post-health shock ($N = 1,796$), activities of daily living limitation (1,406), instrumental activities of daily living limitation (1,070), and cognitive status (1,510) were appreciably lower since we required information from NLTCS interviews both before and after the health shock in such analyses (for example, the prior community resident status in the case of probability of residing in the community after a health shock). Thus, we did not have complete information on any person who died before the next NLTCS wave.

To assess differences in performance by ownership, we classified hospitals into five mutually exclusive categories. First, based on the hospital's intern- and resident-to-bed ratio in the year in which the patient was admitted, we distinguished between teaching and nonteaching hospitals. Second, for hospitals with no residents, and hence no teaching activity, we distinguished between for-profit, government, and private nonprofit hospitals. Teaching is extremely rare among for-profit hospitals.[9] Third, we distinguished between minor teaching and major teaching hospitals. We classified such hospitals on the basis of whether or not the resident-to-bed ratio in the year the beneficiary was admitted was below or above the median ratio (0.097 residents per hospital bed set up and staffed according to AHA data using all hospitals with an index admission that had nonzero residents and interns per bed). We did not distinguish ownership by teaching hospital category. Medicare has used the ratio of interns and residents per bed as a measure of teaching intensity for purposes of subsidizing teaching hospitals (Iglehart 1998).[10]

By category, our sample included 226 persons with an index admission at a nonteaching for-profit hospital. For the other hospital type groups, sample sizes were 416 persons with index admissions in nonteaching government, 1,197 in nonteaching private nonprofit, 421 in minor teaching, and 414 in major teaching hospitals. Among these were 138 for-profit, 163 public, 613 nonprofit, and 243 minor and 221 major teaching hospitals. Assignment of ownership and teaching status was based on the status at the date of the index admission; hence some hospitals changed classifications across study years.

III. Empirical Specification

Dependent Variables

For our analysis of Medicare payments, we specified three dependent variables with the Medicare beneficiary admitted for one of the four conditions as the observational unit: (1) total Medicare payments during the first six months after the index event, (2) total Medicare payments during the first six months less Medicare payments to the first hospital to which the beneficiary was admitted, and (3) total Medicare payments *per week* during the first six months following the index event. All monetarily expressed variables were converted to 1994 dollars using the Consumer Price Index, all items.

One may expect payments for the index inpatient stays for a particular category of beneficiaries to vary for several reasons: hospital coding practices; differences in input prices; explicit subsidies for these hospitals taking a disproportionate share of Medicare and Medicaid patients, graduate medical education, and for capital; and patient use of services excluded from Medicare's fixed price, such as for rehabilitation or psychiatric care in a "distinct part unit." In addition to the regression analysis, we computed means and standard deviations by component of payment.

The second dependent variable was analyzed to study the impact of initial hospitalization on payments not covered by Medicare Prospective Payment for the index admission, including payments for post-acute care. Some hospitals may offer more intensive care that produces savings in care, such as lower rehospitalization rates or institutional care, following discharge from the first hospital. Alternatively, such hospitals may not offer higher intensity, but rather may refer patients to providers with which they have formal or informal contractual relationships, thus raising Medicare payments after discharge.

When beneficiaries survived for 26 weeks, the third dependent variable was only the first dependent variable divided by 26. However, many beneficiaries did not survive the first six months. In such cases, we calculated the length of time (in weeks) from the index admission to the date of death. Total Medicare payments over the same period were then divided by the number of weeks to construct the third dependent variable.

To measure weeks to death and to readmission to a hospital with the same diagnoses, we estimated hazard models with time to failure, death, or readmission, measured in weeks. We assessed mortality separately and jointly with rehospitalization using a competing risks approach, in both cases with Cox proportional hazards models. To gauge whether some types of hospitals were more successful in keeping patients out of nursing homes, we specified a binary dependent variable equal to 1 if the beneficiary lived outside of a nursing home, that is, in the community at the NLTCS interview following the index health hospital stay (either in 1989 or 1994). We included a variable for the person's living arrangement at the NLTCS interview before the index hospitalization (either in 1984 or 1989) as an explanatory variable. Thus, our analysis assessed the extent to which the index health event, ownership of the hospital to which the patient was initially admitted, and other factors affected living arrangements.

Similarly, to investigate changes in functional status from the date of the NLTCS interview before the index event to date of the interview after this event, we specified equations with three dependent variables relating to the respondents' functional status subsequent to the health event: number of dependencies in ADLs and IADLs; and four-point scales representing the degree of difficulty the beneficiary had in climbing a flight of stairs, picking up a ten-pound package and holding it for a few minutes, and using fingers to pick up a small object, such as a dime. The final three measures of functional status are not reflected in the ADL and IADL scales. Difficulty of performing a task was measured on a four-point scale: can't do at all (4); very difficult to do (3); somewhat difficult (2); and not difficult (1).

To assess mental status, we estimated an equation with a binary variable to represent cognitive functioning. We used the ten-question Short Portable Mental Status Questionnaire administered as part of the NLTCS interview as a measure of cognitive status (Pfeiffer 1975). We considered a person to be "cognitively aware" if he or she answered seven or more questions correctly. Questions dealt with orientation in time ("What is today's date?") and place ("What is the name of this place?") and ability to perform simple calculations ("Count backward in threes starting with 20"). Otherwise, or if a proxy respondent was used, this binary was set equal to 0.

Ownership

Our analysis focused on the role of ownership of the hospital to which the beneficiary was first admitted. We used the five categories described above, with for-profit nonteaching hospitals as the omitted reference group.

Other Explanatory Variables

Other explanatory variables fell into four categories: demographic and income; health pre-index hospitalization; primary diagnosis at index hospitalization; and other.

Demographic variables were age at the date of the index hospitalization, gender, years of schooling completed, race (white versus all nonwhite), being married at the NLTCS interview before the index event, and a binary variable indicating beneficiaries first screened after 1984 ("new cohort"). We also included a variable for total household income at the NLTCS interview before the index event.

Included in the prior health category was a binary variable indicating whether the person lived in the community (versus a nursing home), number of ADL limitations, whether or not the person was cognitively aware, and a binary for lack of bowel and/or bladder control, all as reported at the NLTCS full interview or screener before the event occurred. As noted above, the analysis of functional and cognitive status included lagged values of the dependent variable.

For primary diagnosis at index admission, we included a risk adjuster ("comorbidity index") used by Medicare and others to forecast future payments on behalf of the individual (DxCG 1996; Ellis et al. 1996). The comorbidity index classified patients based on age, sex, and diagnoses information contained in the index admission hospital claims record. Diagnoses other than the primary reason for the index admission were reflected in this comorbidity score. This risk classification approach has been used to group Medicare beneficiaries in terms of expected future use of personal health care.

We also included binary variables to account for heterogeneity among primary diagnoses within the four broad diagnostic categories. For stroke, we distinguished between hemorrhagic and ischemic strokes. Likewise, for coronary heart disease, separate binary variables were specified for heart attacks, angina pectoris/unstable angina, and other ischemic heart disease. For congestive heart failure, we distinguished between congestive heart failure that was not associated with another underlying ailment as the primary diagnosis ("uncomplicated congestive heart failure") and congestive heart failure that was associated with renal disease and/or hypertension ("congestive heart failure with renal/hypertensive disease"). For hip fractures, we distinguished between pertrochanteric hip fractures and other fractures, which included transcervical fractures and unspecified hip fracture locations, the former being the omitted reference group.

Other explanatory variables were a variable for the year in which the index event occurred ("time"), the number of years between the year of the index shock and the next NLTCS interview ("NLTCS year"), and population per square mile in the Primary Sampling Unit in which the person resided (Standard Metropolitan Statistical Areas for persons in metropolitan areas and counties for persons living in nonmetropolitan areas). The rationale for including the NLTCS year was that outcomes measured after the index event plausibly reflect time elapsed between the event and the interview. Thus, in general, outcomes should be worse if the interview occurred soon after the index event. Likewise, the information from the NLTCS interview before the index event should be relatively imprecise in such cases.

Analysis of Rehabilitation

Before 1991 Medicare claims data did not permit one to completely determine which beneficiaries received rehabilitative services following the index admission (admissions to inpatient rehabilitation units within hospitals can be identified). From 1991 on, the file included an explicit data element for rehabilitation cost. Rehabilitation may have taken place in a distinct part unit of the index hospital, another rehabilitation hospital, a skilled nursing facility, and/or have been performed by a home health agency.

In our analysis, the dependent variable was 1 if the patient had some form of rehabilitation within one year following the index event and was 0 otherwise. We limited the analysis to index events occurring in 1991 and thereafter. We estimated separate regressions for (1) hip fracture and stroke and (2) the other two diagnoses. Rehabilitation is far more commonly performed for the former than for the latter diagnoses.

Estimation

Because the payment variables were right-skewed, it is important that the functional form selected for analysis reflect this. To account for this, we partitioned the payment variables into quintiles and estimated payment equations using ordered logit analysis. As specified, the total payment quintile distribution was defined by the following maximum values: $4,202; $6,801; $10,888; $17,724; and $104,182, showing a large range for the top quintile. All dollar-valued variables were updated to 1994 dollars, using the Consumer Price Index, all items. The other two payment dependent variables showed a similar type of distribution.

For mortality and rehospitalization, we used the Cox proportional hazard model, with and without a competing risks adjustment. For the rest of the analysis, we used logit or ordered logit, depending on whether the dependent variable was a simple binary or an ordered variable.

IV. Empirical Results

Characteristics of Medicare Beneficiaries Hospitalized by Hospital Category

We compared characteristics of beneficiaries by the ownership and teaching status of the facility to which they were admitted for the index hospitalization (table 5.1). We conducted pairwise t-tests for differences in means, all relative to nonteaching for-profit hospitals. For the vast majority of pairwise comparisons, there were no statistically significant differences.

On demographic variables, mean educational attainment was low for this cohort, but beneficiaries who went to private nonprofit and teaching hospitals tended to have had somewhat more schooling. On income, beneficiaries admitted to major teaching hospitals tended to be more affluent than those admitted to for-profit hospitals. There was only one statistically significant difference in the health of beneficiaries at the NLTCS interview before the index event.

Beneficiaries admitted to government hospitals were less likely to have reported problems with lack of bladder or bowel control before the index admission than were beneficiaries admitted to for-profit hospitals. There were virtually no differences in the distribution of primary diagnosis at the index admission. Most importantly, there were no statistically significant differences in the comorbidity index. This index is based on ICD-9 codes, not DRGs. So if the lack of difference was due to upcoding to increase Medicare payment, the effect would have to have been quite indirect. Measured in terms of population density, the government hospitals in our sample tended to be more rural and the teaching hospitals more urban than were the for-profit hospitals.

Medicare Payments

Overall, for these four diagnoses, total Medicare payments for the first six months following the index admission ranged from $9,100 for government to $15,100 for major teaching hospitals (table 5.2). Total payments made on behalf of beneficiaries who went for their index admission to for-profit and private nonprofit hospitals were almost identical. Payments for both ownership categories exceeded those for beneficiaries admitted to government facilities by $2,500 to $2,900.

Our analysis of spending components was limited by the amount of disaggregation on the Medicare claims files that was possible for the entire period, 1984–95. The basic payment reflected the fixed payment for the index hospitalization, which was based on the DRG assigned to the index admission and the wage index then applicable to the hospital. Added to this were any supplemental payments for outliers. For the four disease categories, we found no statistically significant differences by ownership in the DRG weight assigned to these cases, using the DRG weights for 1995.

Payments outside of the Prospective Payment System (PPS) represented cost-based reimbursement for stays in distinct-part psychiatric, rehabilitation, and swing bed units through 1995, and alcohol units through October 1987. For 1991–95, this category also included cost-based payments for primary care hospitals. There were no statistically significant differences in the means between for-profit and the other ownership types for payments outside of PPS for the index admission.

Major teaching hospitals received much higher amounts of indirect medical education payments (IME) than other hospitals. The small amounts of IME payments that nonteaching facilities received appear to be due to errors in the claims data.[11] Very few such facilities were reported to have received IME payments, and such payments to these facilities were mostly recorded for admissions occurring before 1991.

Spending on home health care on behalf of patients admitted to for-profit hospitals was higher than for all of the other categories. Similarly, spending on physicians' services was higher for the beneficiaries admitted to for-profit facilities compared to all but major teaching hospitals, but none of the mean values were significantly different from the for-profit group at conventional levels of statistical significance.

Adjusting for other determinants of Medicare payments per beneficiary, some differences in payments by ownership remained (table 5.3). Compared to the for-profit facilities, total payments on behalf of beneficiaries admitted to government hospitals were lower; however, those for beneficiaries admitted to major teaching facilities were higher.

Excluding payments for the index admission, beneficiaries admitted to for-profit facilities were more costly to Medicare. Compared to

Table 5.1 Sample Characteristics by Hospital Type

	Means and Standard Deviations									
	For-Profit		Government		Nonprofit		Minor Teaching		Major Teaching	
Demographic/Income										
Age	80.60	(7.28)	80.63	(7.55)	80.60	(7.82)	80.28	(7.96)	79.74	(8.16)
Male	0.28	(0.45)	0.32	(0.47)	0.29	(0.45)	0.27	(0.44)	0.29	(0.46)
Education	8.66	(3.27)	8.61	(3.28)	9.44[a]	(3.20)	9.43[a]	(3.66)	9.73[a]	(3.13)
White	0.92	(0.28)	0.90	(0.30)	0.91	(0.29)	0.88	(0.33)	0.87[c]	(0.34)
Married	0.33	(0.47)	0.39	(0.49)	0.39[c]	(0.49)	0.35	(0.48)	0.33	(0.47)
New Cohort	0.027	(0.16)	0.031	(0.17)	0.038	(0.19)	0.033	(0.18)	0.039	(0.19)
Income ('000)	1.55	(1.23)	0.51	(1.24)	1.73[c]	(1.36)	1.74[c]	(1.28)	1.91[a]	(1.59)
Health, Pre-Index Admission										
Lived in community	0.84	(0.37)	0.81	(0.39)	0.83	(0.37)	0.81	(0.39)	0.84	(0.36)
No. ADLs	1.56	(2.00)	1.82	(2.15)	1.68	(2.08)	1.83	(2.07)	1.55	(2.041)
Cognitively aware	0.36	(0.48)	0.39	(0.49)	0.41	(0.49)	0.38	(0.49)	0.43[c]	(0.50)
Lack bowel/bladder control	0.071	(0.26)	0.029[b]	(0.17)	0.044	(0.21)	0.048	(0.21)	0.051	(0.22)

Primary Diagnosis at Index Admission										
Comorbidity index	0.65	(1.27)	0.60	(1.39)	0.68	(1.25)	0.67	(1.38)	0.59	(1.17)
Hemorrhaghic stroke	0.022	(0.15)	0.031	(0.17)	0.033	(0.18)	0.036	(0.19)	0.027	(0.16)
Ischemic stroke	0.26	(0.44)	0.24	(0.43)	0.22	(0.41)	0.23	(0.42)	0.22	(0.42)
Other hip fracture	0.13	(0.34)	0.13	(0.33)	0.13	(0.34)	0.12	(0.32)	0.11	(0.31)
Petrochateric hip fracture	0.13	(0.34)	0.13	(0.33)	0.18[b]	(0.38)	0.15	(0.35)	0.16	(0.36)
Congestive heart failure	0.15	(0.36)	0.17	(0.37)	0.16	(0.37)	0.14	(0.35)	0.13	(0.33)
Cong. heart failure/other	0.018	(0.13)	0.017	(0.13)	0.014	(0.12)	0.012	(0.11)	0.012	(0.11)
Heart attack	0.12	(0.32)	0.11	(0.31)	0.10	(0.30)	0.12	(0.33)	0.14	(0.35)
Angina pectoris/unstable	0.15	(0.35)	0.16	(0.36)	0.13	(0.34)	0.14	(0.35)	0.14	(0.35)
Ischemic heart disease	0.027	(0.16)	0.029	(0.17)	0.030	(0.17)	0.052[c]	(0.22)	0.065[b]	(0.25)
Other										
Time	4.45	(2.60)	4.00[b]	(2.43)	4.36	(2.62)	3.74	(2.54)	4.16	(2.54)
NLTCS year	1.68	(1.35)	1.75	(1.36)	1.68	(1.38)	1.48	(1.40)	1.76	(1.47)
Population density (0000)	0.62	(0.99)	0.19[a]	(0.33)	0.57	(0.82)	0.78[b]	(0.94)	1.30[a]	(1.33)
N	226		416		1,197		421		414	

NOTE: $^{a}p \leq .01$; $^{b}p \leq .05$; $^{c}p \leq .10$

Reference group is for-profit hospitals.

Table 5.2 Mean Medicare Payments by Hospital Type (1994$)

	For-Profit	Government	Nonprofit	Minor Teaching	Major Teaching
DRG + Factor Price	5,620	4,413[a]	5,850	6,350[c]	7,236[a]
Capital/DME	127	75[a]	113	107	159
DSH	37	31	36	51	113[a]
IME	4	22[b]	30[a]	106[a]	390[a]
Payment Outside of PPS	313	164	224	466	156
Total Index	6,101	4,706[a]	6,254	7,081[b]	8,054[a]
Total Rehospitalization	2,497	2,067	2,454	2,410	3,784[b]
Part B Physician	1,676	1,115[a]	1,420	1,434	1,735
Outpatient	337	245	292	299	399
Home Health	710	491[c]	491[c]	403[b]	458[b]
SNF	606	448[a]	701	644	714
Hospice	0	3	0	2	0
Total 6 Months	11,927	9,075[a]	11,611	12,273	15,145[a]
N	226	416	1,197	421	414

NOTE: [a]$p \leq .01$; [b]$p \leq .05$; [c]$p \leq .10$

KEY: DME = direct medical education; DSH = disproportionate share hospital; IME = indirect medical education; SNF = skilled nursing facility

those who went to for-profit hospitals, payments for patients hospitalized in government hospitals were 5 percent less likely to be in the top quintile of the payment distribution. Payments were also lower for those who went to nonprofit hospitals.

Expressing total Medicare payments on a weekly basis somewhat compressed payment differentials by ownership. Again payments were lower for patients admitted to government compared to for-profit facilities. Many of the explanatory variables other than hospital ownership were statistically significant at conventional levels but are not shown in the table to conserve space.[12]

In table 5.4, we show the probabilities of being in a particular quintile of the distribution of payments made by Medicare on behalf of Medicare beneficiaries during the first six months following the index event. Not adjusting for covariates other than ownership-teaching, payments to government hospitals were 0.16 more likely to be in the

Table 5.3 Effects of Ownership on Medicare Payments, Other Payment Determinants Held Constant

	Ordered Logit Regression							
	Total First 6 months		Total 6 Months Less Index			Total Weekly First 6 Months		
	Coeff.	(s.e.)	Coeff.	(s.e.)	[m.e.]	Coeff.	(s.e.)	[m.e.]
Government	−0.60[a]	(0.15)	−0.34[b]	(0.15)	[−0.05]	−0.25[c]	(0.15)	[−0.04]
Nonprofit	−0.20	(0.13)	−0.26[b]	(0.13)	[−0.04]	−0.065	(0.13)	[−0.01]
Minor Teaching	0.0059	(0.15)	−0.28[b]	(0.15)	[−0.04]	0.017	(0.15)	[0.00]
Major Teaching	0.32[b]	(0.15)	−0.070	(0.15)	[−0.01]	0.22	(0.16)	[0.03]

NOTE: [a]p ≤ .01; [b]p ≤ .05; [c]p ≤ .10

Significance tests indicate the underlying regression coefficient was significantly different from 0.

Hospital types are relative to for-profit hospitals, controlling for demographic factors, preshock health status, primary diagnosis, year of index even, and population density.

Marginal effects are for the probability of being in the highest payment quintile for the dependent variable. Marginal effects for the total first six months are shown in table 5.4.

Table 5.4 Marginal Effects of Ownership on Total Medicare Payments

	Total Payment Quintile				
	1	2	3	4	5
A. Unadjusted					
Government	0.16	0.00	−0.01	−0.07	−0.08
Nonprofit	0.02	0.02	−0.01	−0.02	−0.01
Minor Teaching	0.00	0.00	0.00	−0.03	0.03
Major Teaching	−0.06	−0.04	−0.02	0.02	0.10
B. Adjusted					
Government	0.09	0.06	−0.00	−0.06	−0.08
Nonprofit	0.03	0.02	−0.00	−0.02	−0.03
Minor Teaching	−0.00	−0.00	0.00	0.00	0.00
Major Teaching	−0.05	−0.03	0.00	0.03	0.04

NOTE: Adjusted marginal effects are from the ordered logit analysis reported in table 5.3.

Payment quintile 1 is the lowest; 5 is the highest.

lowest quintile and 0.08 less likely to be in the highest quintile than were for-profits. At the other end of the spectrum, major teaching hospitals were 0.06 less likely to be in the lowest quintile and 0.10 more likely to be than in highest-quintile for-profit facilities. The pattern of results is basically unchanged when adjustments are made for the other covariates. However, the differences by hospital type are somewhat smaller.

Mortality

Of the 2,674 patients studied, 1,924 (72.0 percent) died between an index admission for a study condition and December 31, 1995. Figure 5.1 shows Kaplan-Meier plots of crude mortality differences by hospital type. Patients admitted to major teaching hospitals had appreciably higher survival rates, even at four years following the index admission. The lowest rate of survival was for nonteaching government hospitals. The relative performance of such hospitals was maintained not only initially but throughout the four-year period following the index admissions. For-profit hospitals had the second lowest survival rates up to two years after the index event. Subsequently, survival for patients initially admitted to for-profit hospitals was indistinguishable from experience of patients admitted to nonteaching nonprofit and minor teaching hospitals. The Kaplan-Meier technique accounts for censoring by projecting survival based on trends that are observed. Thus, because an increasing number of cases are censored as time from the index admission elapsed, survival rates shown for the first two years following the index admission are more reliable than for the subsequent two years.

The data shown in figure 5.1 do not hold other determinants of survival other than hospital ownership, such as case-mix severity, constant. Using a hazard model that accounted for the effects of other factors, survival was much better for patients admitted to major teaching hospitals than for those admitted to for-profit hospitals (HR = hazard ratio of dying after admission to major teaching hospital relative to for-profit, 0.76, $p = 0.01$) (table 5.5, column 1).[13] For-profit hospitals were found to have the worst mortality of any hospital type when adjusting for patient characteristics, but the differences between for-profit hospital mortality and mortality in government, not-for-profit, and minor teaching hospitals were not statistically significant at conventional levels.

We also estimated a hazard model that accounted for competing

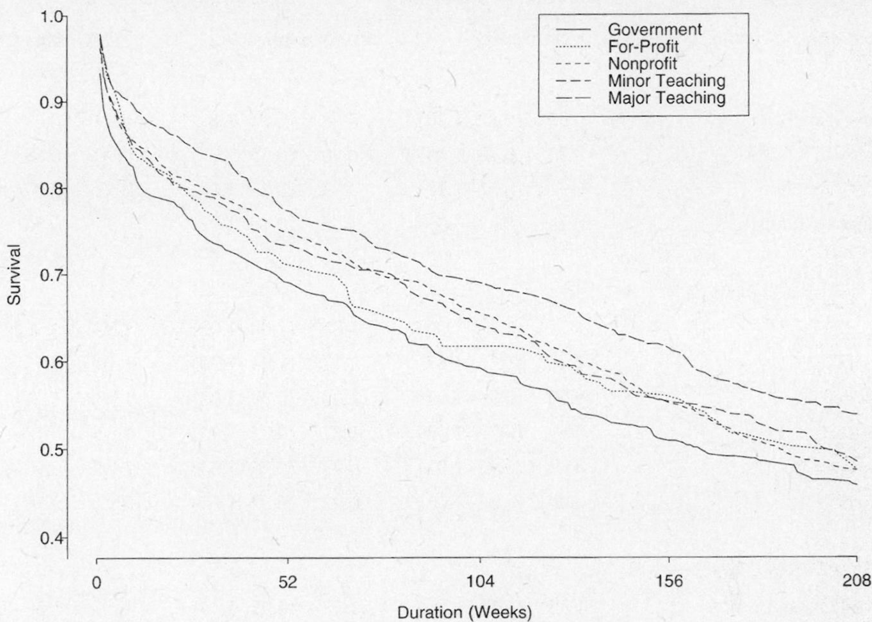

Figure 5.1 Crude Survival Differences by Hospital Type, from Index Admission through Four Years

risks, rehospitalization, and mortality, simultaneously. Of the total deaths observed, 34 percent died before being readmitted for the same diagnosis. The major change when accounting for the competing risks of rehospitalization and mortality is that the improved survival of major teaching hospitals is no longer statistically significant at conventional levels ($p = 0.11$) and the time trend for mortality becomes negative and highly significant, implying a reduction in the probability of dying before readmission over time.

Many of the other coefficients are plausible and statistically significant: age ($HR = 1.05$); number of ADLs before the shock ($HR = 1.23$); and several variables for primary diagnosis at index admission, including hemorrhagic stroke ($HR = 1.86$), ischemic stroke ($HR = 1.58$), congestive heart failure ($HR = 1.82$), and heart attack ($HR = 1.55$). Two statistically significant findings—having lived in the community ($HR = 1.35$) and having been cognitively aware ($HR = 1.30$), all defined before the health shock—seem implausible at first glance.

Deaths occurring before the person arrived at a hospital for an index admission were excluded from our sample. To further investigate the

Table 5.5 Mortality and Rehospitalization Using Cox Proportional Hazards Model

Explanatory Variables	Without Competing Risks		Competing Risks Model			
	Mortality		Rehospitalization		Mortality	
Ownership						
Government	0.99	(0.82–1.20)	0.98	(0.81–1.19)	0.99	(0.69–1.35)
Nonprofit	0.93	(0.78–1.09)	0.90	(0.75–1.07)	0.90	(0.68–1.22)
Minor teaching	0.91	(0.75–1.10)	0.89	(0.73–1.08)	0.92	(0.67–1.26)
Major teaching	0.76[a]	(0.63–0.93)	1.00	(0.83–1.22)	0.75	(0.53–1.08)
Demographic/Income						
Age	1.05[a]	(1.05–1.06)	1.01[b]	(1.00–1.02)	1.07[a]	(1.06–1.08)
Male	1.42[a]	(1.26–1.57)	1.17[a]	(1.04–1.30)	1.14	(0.95–1.40)
Education	1.00	(0.99–1.01)	1.00	(0.99–1.02)	1.03[b]	(1.01–1.05)
White	0.89	(0.77–1.04)	0.87[c]	(0.75–1.02)	1.05	(0.78–1.41)
Income ('000)	0.99	(0.95–1.02)	0.99	(0.95–1.03)	1.01	(0.96–1.08)
Married	0.96	(0.86–1.08)	0.92	(0.82–1.04)	0.93	(0.76–1.12)
Health, Pre-Index Admission						
Lived in community	1.35[a]	(1.14–1.59)	1.18[c]	(0.97–1.44)	1.67[a]	(1.30–2.17)
No. ADLs	1.23[a]	(1.20–1.27)	1.04[b]	(1.01–1.08)	1.27[a]	(1.21–1.34)
Cognitively aware	1.30[a]	(1.18–1.42)	1.10[c]	(1.00–1.22)	1.24[a]	(1.06–1.47)
Lack bowel/bladder control	1.17	(0.94–1.44)	1.13	(0.91–1.40)	0.82	(0.51–1.25)
Primary Diagnosis at Index Admission						
Comorbidity index	1.09[a]	(1.05 –1.13)	1.04[c]	(1.00–1.08)	1.15[a]	(1.07–1.21)
Hemorrhagic stroke	1.86[a]	(1.41–2.45)	1.07	(0.75–1.51)	3.31[a]	(2.20–4.82)
Ischemic stroke	1.58[a]	(1.36–1.84)	1.22[b]	(1.02–1.43)	2.17[a]	(1.69–2.71)
Other hip fracture	1.04	(0.88–1.24)	0.86	(0.72–1.05)	1.12	(0.85–1.47)
Congestive heart failure	1.82[a]	(1.55–2.14)	2.07[a]	(1.73–2.44)	1.69[a]	(1.25–2.26)
CHF with renal/hyper	1.95[a]	(1.32–2.89)	1.86[a]	(1.24–2.78)	1.90	(0.82–4.41)
Heart attack	1.55[a]	(1.29–1.86)	1.70[a]	(1.38–2.05)	3.01[a]	(2.22–3.99)
Angina pectoris/unstable	0.84[c]	(0.70–1.02)	1.51[a]	(1.26–1.80)	0.37[a]	(0.22–0.63)
Ischemic heart disease	0.84	(0.61–1.14)	1.59[a]	(1.22–2.02)	0.70	(0.34–1.44)
Other						
Time	1.01	(1.01–1.03)	0.94[a]	(0.93–0.97)	0.94[a]	(0.93–0.99)
Population density	1.01	(0.97–1.07)	0.98	(0.93–1.03)	0.99	(0.91–1.08)
N	2,674		2,674		2,674	
N failures	1,924		1,766		653	

NOTE: [a]p ≤ .01; [b]p ≤ .05; [c]p ≤ .10

Cox models were estimated using SAS; competing risks assumes death and readmission are statistically independent. Failures for competing risk mortality signifies deaths before readmission.

selection process results, we specified a logistic regression model of all deaths occurring among NLTCS respondents from 1984 through 1995 that were not included in our study sample; 1 was for deaths that occurred in the hospital and 0 for deaths at other sites. This analysis indicated that persons living in the community at the NLTCS prior to their death were more likely to die in a hospital, as were those living in more urban areas. Those with greater ADL limitations prior to the index event were less likely to die in a hospital, as were those with a higher comorbidity index score calculated using all ICD-9-CM information from all Medicare files prior to death. However, those who were cognitively aware at the NLTCS prior to death were found to be more likely to die in a hospital, but this result was not statistically significant at conventional levels. These results are suggestive of a pattern of more aggressive treatment of a health shock for those with higher baseline health status.

Rehospitalization

We found no statistically significant differences by ownership of the hospital at which the patient had an index admission on time to rehospitalization for the primary diagnosis for which a study subject was first admitted (table 5.5, column 2). There was a negative time trend that was highly significant ($p = 0.01$), suggesting a reduced likelihood of being readmitted over time.

Living in the Community after the Health Shock

We found no statistically significant differences in the probability of being in the community as opposed to a nursing home at the NLTCS interview following the index health event between patients admitted to for-profit versus the other types of hospitals (table 5.6). These findings were not sensitive to changes in equation specification. Interestingly, patients admitted to major teaching hospitals had the highest probability of living in the community at the time of the NLTCS interview following the health event.

Functional and Cognitive Status

Our results from ordered logit analysis of activities of daily living (ADL) and instrumental activities of daily living (IADL) and logit

Table 5.6 Living in Community, Functional Status, and Cognitive Status at Next NLTCS Survey

	Marginal Effects				
Outcome Measures	**Government**	**Nonprofit**	**Minor Teaching**	**Major Teaching**	***N***
Community residence	−0.029	−0.029	−0.023	0.060	1,796
Activities of daily living (ADLs)	−0.039	−0.013	0.019	0.054	1,406
Instrumental activities of daily living (IADLs)	−0.066	−0.092[c]	−0.10[c]	0.010	1,070
Cognitively aware	−0.057	−0.034	−0.071	−0.000015	1,510
Climb flight of stairs	−0.058[c]	0.0044	−0.046	0.0034	712
Lift 10 lbs. above head	0.071	0.085[b]	−0.0097	−0.086[c]	761
Grasp small objects with fingers	0.084	0.12[b]	0.072	0.15[b]	783

NOTE: [a]$p \leq .01$; [b]$p \leq .05$; [c]$p \leq .10$

Marginal effects for ordered logit analysis are calculated in the case where the dependent variable is equal to 0 (no limitations; highest functioning).

analysis of being cognitively aware at the postevent interview date were consistent with those from our logit analysis of being in the community. The changes in the probability for ADL and IADL shown in table 5.6 are for no ADLs or no IADLs versus having some limitations. Thus, relative to beneficiaries admitted to for-profit facilities, those admitted to government hospitals had a 0.039 lower probability of having no ADLs at the NLTCS interview after the index event, holding other factors constant, including the number of ADLs the person had at the NLTCS interview before the event. Patients admitted to major teaching hospitals had a 0.054 higher probability of not having ADLs than those admitted to for-profit hospitals. However, none of these differences were statistically significant at conventional levels.

For having no IADLs, two of the marginal effects were statistically significant at better than the 10 percent level. Both patients of nonprofit and minor teaching hospitals were more likely to have IADL limitations at the NLTCS interview after the index admission.

For cognitive status, holding other factors constant, patients admitted to for-profit hospitals were more likely to be "cognitively aware" at the NLTCS interview after the event than were patients admitted to the other types of facilities. However, none of the effects were statistically significant at conventional levels. The probability for patients at major teaching hospitals was almost identical to that for for-profit facilities.

The ADL and IADL measures did not directly capture variation in cardiovascular fitness or in small motor coordination. Relative to the patients admitted to for-profit hospitals, government hospital patients reported greater difficulty in climbing a flight of steps. In the marginal effects reported in table 5.6, government hospital patients had a 0.058 lower probability of reporting difficulty in climbing steps at the NLTCS interview after the index admission. For the other ownership types, there were no statistically significant differences between for-profit facilities and the other ownership groups. By contrast, for lifting a ten-pound package and holding it for a few minutes and grasping a small object like a dime, patients at for-profit hospitals were less likely to report having no difficulty than those hospitalized at nonprofit or major teaching facilities. The differences in probabilities of having no difficulty were especially substantial for grasping, 0.12 for nonprofit and 0.15 for major teaching hospitals.

Receipt of Rehabilitation Services

We assessed differences in the likelihood of receiving rehabilitation services by hospital type for index admissions occurring on January 1, 1991, and subsequently (table 5.7). None of the differences in probability of receiving such services differed at conventional levels of statistical significance. This pattern held true for hip fracture and stroke, for

Table 5.7 Effect of Hospital Ownership on Receipt of Rehabilitation, 1991 95

	Marginal Effects	
	Stroke/ Hip Fracture	**Coronary Heart Disease/ Congestive Heart Failure**
Government	−0.069	−0.014
Nonprofit	0.0070	0.018
Minor Teaching	−0.17	−0.047
Major Teaching	0.13	−0.10
N	230	311
N Receiving	155 (67%)	84 (24%)

NOTE: $^a p \leq .01$; $^b p \leq .05$; $^c p \leq .10$

Analysis for index admissions occurring 1 January 1991 through 1 July 1995. Marginal effects are for the probability of receiving some rehabilitation care within one year post index admission.

which 67 percent of all patients received some rehabilitation, as well as for coronary heart disease and congestive heart failure, where 24 percent of patients did. Interestingly, patients with an index admission in a major teaching hospital had an increased probability (0.13) of receiving some rehabilitation after stroke or hip fracture, but a lower probability (0.10) of receiving such services after an index admission for coronary heart disease or congestive heart failure, relative to for-profit hospitals.

V. Discussion

Gauged in terms of total Medicare payments after the index event, beneficiaries admitted to for-profit hospitals were more costly than those admitted to public facilities and less costly than those admitted to major teaching hospitals. The differential between for-profit and public hospitals is not explained by significantly improved survival by patients with index admissions in for-profit hospitals relative to public facilities, but is partly due to lower spending on postacute care for patients admitted to the latter facilities. The relative costliness of major teaching facilities was attributable to higher payments for the index admission and readmission, not to differences in payments for physicians' services and for postacute care. Differences in Medicare payments received by different types of hospitals were reduced when a crude adjustment for health outcomes (weekly payment) was used without changing the relative rankings of payments.

Differences in payments other than for the index admission are noteworthy, especially the higher payments for home health care on behalf of patients who had been hospitalized for the index admission at for-profit facilities and payments to physicians for care rendered both in the hospital and on an ambulatory basis. The latter were appreciably higher for patients who had gone to for-profit facilities than they were for patients admitted to other nonteaching hospitals. These differences were not statistically significant at conventional levels because of appreciable variation in such expenditures within hospital ownership categories.

Survival of patients admitted to major teaching hospitals was much better than survival of patients admitted to nonteaching hospitals, irrespective of their ownership. The record for functional and cognitive status of survivors was mixed, sometimes favoring for-profits (IADLs) and sometimes favoring others (two of the three measures of other functioning). However, in the vast majority of cases, the conclusion is one of no difference. This leads to a general conclusion that for these four major sources of morbidity and mortality among the elderly, for-profit hospitals provide about the same quality care as other nonteaching hospitals and cost more than other types of nonteaching hospitals. Major teaching hospitals are the most expensive hospital type but show evidence of better outcomes.

We compared the sample patients by hospital type of index admission using the explanatory variables used in the Medicare payment analysis. We found surprisingly few differences in terms of the characteristics of the patients treated.

To our knowledge, ours is the first study of hospital ownership form to compare performance on the basis of what a single payer paid for care, both at the hospital to which the patient was admitted and downstream. There are two issues. First, what are the implications of using our "cost" measure? Second, to the extent that our results can be compared, how do they differ from those obtained by others?

We used actual Medicare payments for services delivered and not charges in order to approximate cost of care, hospital and otherwise. Medicare payments may vary by ownership for several reasons: competitive advantages conferred by governments; differential provision of public goods; teaching and/or research; slack; quality; and case-mix severity. The core issue, however, for economic research on hospital cost has been to determine whether for-profit hospitals are indeed more efficient. Various methods, including regression and frontier production functions, have been used to compare the efficiency of hospital types (Sloan 1998). Unlike our study, past researchers examined various measures of hospital cost or input use, not program cost, such as Medicare payments. Although the studies have yielded some conflicting findings, overall, the empirical evidence does not demonstrate that for-profit hospitals are more efficient.

The most rigorous and extensive study of quality published to date that permits comparisons of quality by hospital ownership is by Keeler et al. (1992). Like this study, they restricted their research to persons over age 65. They used two measures of the care process based on reviews of 14,000 medical records for five diseases (some of which overlap with ours) in 297 hospitals in five states. They found no difference in quality between private nonprofit and for-profit hospitals on two indicators. Public hospitals fared worse on both criteria. However, on a third measure—mortality within thirty days of admission to the hospital—there was a statistically significant difference between quality of private nonprofits and for-profit and public hospitals. The authors appear to have been more persuaded by the results on the first two indicators, concluding that "nonprofit and for-profit hospitals provide similar quality overall" (p. 1,712). Like us, they consistently found that major teaching hospitals had better quality than nonteaching hospitals, measured by excess mortality and the two other process-related measures.

Finally, what are the implications of this empirical analysis? First, from the standpoint of Medicare, differences in program cost and quality between nonteaching for-profits and nonprofits are, on the whole, minimal with one caveat. In further research not present here, we investigated the endogeneity of hospital ownership type among nonteaching facilities (for-profit, nonprofit, and government) and hospital payments, and found evidence that ownership type was endogenous for this subsample. The practical result was to about double payment differentials between nonprofits and for-profits presented here. For all of the outcome measures, we did not find evidence of endogeneity. The program cost differential between government and for-profit hospitals remained much larger than the one between for-profit and nonprofit hospitals. We did not test for endogeneity of admission to a teaching facility because this would be much harder to do (because of lack of suitable instrumental variables). If anything, treating teaching as endogenous would compress the payment differences, and the outcome differences would be even more favorable to teaching hospitals.

Second, the major question for Medicare relative to major teaching hospitals is to determine whether the social subsidy payments in the form of indirect medical education and disproportionate share payments could be reduced without negatively affecting the mortality benefit we detected when patients were initially admitted to such hospitals. Major teaching facilities cost the Medicare program more for inpatient care, and there is interest in reducing or capping such payments in the future. Social subsidies contribute to roughly 5 percent of the total cost of an index admission, but it is not clear if this level of subsidy is partly responsible for the mortality advantage we detected. Improved mortality is a societal benefit that should be carefully weighed when discussing a reduction in Medicare subsidy of the teaching and indigent care mission of such hospitals.

Third, the rapid rise of postacute services financed by Medicare, including rehabilitation, is a major policy area for future consideration (Medicare Payment Advisory Commission 1998). Our results show that the type of hospital to which a Medicare beneficiary is initially admitted has an important impact on the cost of care to Medicare delivered after the index admission. Total mean payments made on behalf of patients admitted to for-profit hospitals were more similar to major teaching facilities than were other nonteaching hospital types, and patients initially admitted into for-profit facilities had the highest payments after the index admission. Our study did not investigate contractual or informal relationships that for-profit hospitals may have had with non-hospital providers, which may explain post index admission payments differentials.

Payment for postacute services such as rehabilitation is moving toward prospective payment with all rehabilitation providers to be reimbursed in this manner by the year 2000 (Medicare Payment Advisory Commission 1998). In addition, further oversight of the linkages between hospitals and other providers of such services may be necessary to slow the rate of growth of these services. Such discussions are particularly important since the increased post-index payments made on behalf of patients initially admitted to for-profit hospitals did not result in any detectable quality advantages.

Finally, Medicare seems unlikely to directly enact any controls over patient choice of hospital, a hallmark of the program for its over thirty-year existence. However, the Balanced Budget Act (BBA) of 1997 expands the options for Medicare patients to sign up for private health plans with the goal of trying to harness some of the cost-slowing processes witnessed in the private market over the past few years for the Medicare program. Private insurance plans must offer the same benefits that traditional fee-for-service Medicare offers, and such plans often include others as a marketing strategy, such as prescription drugs. Paradoxically, the BBA of 1997, hailed widely as expanding beneficiary "choice" of health insurance arrangements, may in fact serve to *reduce* their choice of hospital, as most insurance products currently offered in the marketplace (HMO, PPO, and so on) limit the choice of hospital for an insured individual. In this context, our findings suggest that all nonteaching hospitals offer similar quality and that government facilities would appear to represent the "best buy" for such private insurers and for Medicare. Teaching hospitals provide better quality but for a price. As the proportion of Medicare beneficiaries in plans other than traditional fee-for-service increases (in 1997, 13 percent of beneficiaries were in risk plans, accounting for $24 billion in program costs [Medicare Payment Advisory Commission 1998]), Medicare may not have to worry about restricting choice to lower-cost hospitals. Rather, such channeling will occur on a market-by-market basis through the negotiations between insurers and hospitals. Patients, by choosing particular insurance arrangements outside of the traditional fee-for-service benefit, may do the job for Medicare.

Notes

1. See generally Hansmann (1996).
2. This point is discussed in greater length in Sloan (1988).
3. See Prospective Payment Assessment Commission (1997), p. 71.
4. The Physician Payment Review Commission (1997, 383–86) discussed three reasons for special support for teaching hospitals: (1) ensure beneficiary access to teaching hospitals, (2) ensure the viability of teaching hospitals, and/or (3) support the training of physicians to meet Medicare beneficiaries' needs.
5. Explicit costs of research are not covered by Medicare. Holding a large number of other factors constant, costs of care in teaching hospitals have been reported to be higher. See, for example, Sloan et al. (1983), Garber et al. (1984), Sloan and Valvona (1986), Welch (1987), Thorpe (1988), Iezzoni et al. (1990), Zimmerman et al. 1993), and Custer and Willke (1991).
6. See Gray and Schlesinger (1997), Kuttner (1996a, 1996b, 1997), and Sloan et al. (1997).
7. Both ADLs and IADLs, especially the former, have been shown to predict nursing home use and mortality among the elderly (Svensson et al. 1996; Wolinsky et al. 1997).
8. The ICD-9-CM codes used to select the sample were hip fracture—820, 820.0, 8.208–.209, 820.00, 820.2–.3; 820.11, 820.8x, 820.09–.10, 820.12–.13, 820.19–.22, 820.30–.31; stroke—430–32, 431.9, 432.0, 432.1, 432.9, 434, 434.0, 434.1, 434.9, 436, 436.0, 436.00, 436.34; coronary heart disease—410.0–.9, 411.1, 411.8–.81, 411.89, 413.0–.9, 414.0–.05, 414.8–.9; or congestive heart failure—398.91, 402.01, 402.11, 402.91, 404.01, 404.03, 404.11, 404.13, 404.91, 404.93, 428.0–.1, 428.9.
9. Two hundred twenty-six (87.2 percent) of the for-profit hospitals in our sample were not teaching hospitals. Thirty-two (12.4 percent) were minor teaching hospitals, and one (0.4 percent) was classified as a major teaching hospital. Nonprofits represented 85.5 percent and 86.5 percent of the major and minor teaching hospitals in our sample, respectively; the remainder were government hospitals.
10. Different thresholds have been used in past research. For example, Keeler et al. (1992) used a threshold ratio of 0.062 to distinguish between hospitals with a limited role in teaching from teaching facilities with a moderate role, and a threshold of 0.27 and greater to identify major teaching. The Medicare Prospective Pay-

ment Assessment Commission (1997, 69) used a threshold of 0.25 to distinguish major teaching hospitals from other teaching hospitals.

11. We investigated cases where IME payments accrued to hospitals classified as nonteaching by matching Medicare provider numbers to the name of the hospital and then looking up the hospital in the AHA Annual Guide for the year of the index admission. Based on this review, we determined that such payments appear to be due to errors in the claims data and not misclassification of hospitals as nonteaching.

12. Full results are available from the authors upon request.

13. We also estimated hazard models for mortality and rehospitalization that accounted for omitted heterogeneity. Qualitatively, the findings were very similar to those presented here.

References

American Hospital Association. *Annual Statistics: 1995.* Chicago: American Hospital Association.

Chan, L., T. D. Koepsell, R. A. Deyo, et al. 1997. "The Effect of Medicare's Payment System for Rehabilitation Hospitals on Length of Stay, Charges, and Total Payments." *The New England Journal of Medicine* 337: 978–85.

Custer, W. S., and R. J. Willke. 1991. "Teaching Hospital Costs: The Effects of Medical Staff Characteristics." *Health Services Research* 25: 831–57.

DxCG, Inc. 1996. "DxCG Software Version: 02e (Medicare) Program Documentation." Waltham, Mass.: DxCG, Inc.

Ellis, R. P., G. C. Pope, and L. I. Iezzoni et al. 1996. "Diagnosis-Based Risk Adjustment for Medicare Capitation Payments. *Health Care Financing Review* 17: 101–128.

Garber, A. M., V. R. Fuchs, and J. F. Silverman. 1984. "Case Mix, Costs, and Outcomes: Differences between Faculty and Community Services in a University Hospital." *The New England Journal of Medicine* 310: 1,231–37.

Gray, B., and M. Schlesinger. 1997. "The Profit Transformation of the Hospital and HMO Fields." Unpublished manuscript.

Hansmann, H. 1996. *The Ownership of Enterprise*. Cambridge: Belknap Press of Harvard University Press.

Iezzoni, L. I., M. Shwartz, M. A. Moskowitz, A. S. Ash, E. Sawitz, and S. Burnside. 1990. "Illness Severity and Costs of Admissions at Teaching and Nonteaching Hospitals." *Journal of the American Medical Association* 264: 1,426–31.

Iglehart, J. K. 1998. "Medicare and Graduate Medical Education." *The New England Journal of Medicine* 338: 402–407.

Institute of Medicine. 1986. *For-Profit Enterprise in Health Care*. Washington, D.C.: National Academy Press.

Katz, S., and A. Akpo. 1976. "A Measure of Primary Sociobiological Functions." *International Journal of Health Services* 6: 493–508.

Keeler, E. B., L. V. Rubenstein, K. I. Kahn, D. Draper, E. R. Harrison, M. J.

Mcginty, W. H. Rogers, and R. H. Brook. 1992. "Hospital Characteristics and Quality of Care." *Journal of the American Medical Association* 268: 1,709–14.

Kramer, A. M., J. R. Steiner, R. E. Schlenker et al. 1997. "Outcomes and Costs after Hip Fracture and Stroke: A Comparison of Rehabilitation Settings." *Journal of the American Medical Association* 277: 396–404.

Kuttner, R. 1996a. "Columbia/HCA and the Resurgence of the For-Profit Hospital Business (First of Two Parts)." *New England Journal of Medicine* 335: 362–67.

———. 1996b. "Columbia/HCA and the Resurgence of the For-Profit Hospital Business (Second of Two Parts)." *New England Journal of Medicine* 335: 446–51.

———. 1997. *Everything for Sale*. New York: Alfred A. Knopf.

Lave, J. R. 1985. *The Medicare Adjustment for the Indirect Costs of Medical Education, Historical Development, and Current Status.* American Association of Medical Colleges.

Manton, K. G., and E. Stallard. 1991. "Cross-sectional Estimates of Active Life Expectancy for the U.S. Elderly and Oldest-Old Population." *Journal of Gerontology and Social Sciences* 46: S170–182.

Manton, K. G., E. Stallard, and L. Corder. 1995. "Changes in Morbidity and Chronic Disability in the U.S. Elderly Population: Evidence from the 1982, 1984, and 1989 National Long-Term Care Surveys." *Journal of Gerontology and Social Sciences* 50B: S194–S204.

Medicare Payment Advisory Commission. 1998. *Report to the Congress: Context for a Changing Medicare Program*. Washington, D.C.: Medicare Payment Advisory Commission.

National Institute on Aging. 1998. *Databases on Aging: Survey Summaries.* Bethesda, Md.: National Institute of Health.

Pfeiffer, E. 1975. "A Short Portable Mental Status Questionnaire for the Assessment of Organic Brain Deficit in Elderly Patients." *Journal of the American Geriatric Society* 23: 433–41.

Physician Payment Review Commission. 1997. *Annual Report to Congress*.

Prospective Payment Assessment Commission. 1997. *Medicare and the American Health Care System: Report to the Congress* (June). Washington, D.C.

Sloan, F. A. 1988. "Property Rights in the Hospital Industry." In *Health Care in America,* edited by H. E. Frech III. San Francisco: Pacific Research Institute for Public Policy, pp. 103–41.

———. 1998. "Not-for-Profit Ownership and Hospital Behavior." In *Handbook of Health Economics*, edited by J. P. Newhouse and A. Culyer. Elsevier Science.

Sloan, F. A., R. D. Feldman, and B. Steinwald. 1983. "Effects of Teaching on Hospital Costs." *Journal of Health Economics* 2: 1–28.

Sloan, F. A., D. H. Taylor, and C. J. Conover. Forthcoming. "Hospital Conversions: Is the Purchase Price Too Low? In *National Bureau of Economic Research,* edited by D. Cutler. Chicago: University of Chicago Press.

Sloan, F. A., and J. Valvona. 1986. "The High Cost of Teaching Hospitals." *Health Affairs* 5: 68–85.

Svensson, O., L. Stromberg, G. Ohlen, and U. Lindgren. 1996. "Prediction of the Outcome after Hip Fracture in Elderly Patients." *Journal of Bone and Joint Surgery* 78-B: 115–18.

Thorpe, K. E. 1988. "Why Are Urban Hospital Costs So High? The Relative Importance of Patient Source of Admission, Teaching, Competition, and Case Mix." *Health Services Research* 22: 821–36.

Welch, W. P. 1987. "Do All Teaching Hospitals Deserve an Add-on Payment Under the Prospective Payment System?" *Inquiry* 24 (fall): 221–32.

Welch, H. G., D. E. Wennber, and H. P. Welch. 1996. "The Use of Medicare Home Health Care Services." *The New England Journal of Medicine* 335: 324–29.

Wolinsky, F. D., J. F. Fitzgerald, and T. E. Stump. 1997. "The Effect of Hip Fracture on Mortality, Hospitalization, and Functional Status: A Prospective Study." *American Journal of Public Health* 87: 398–403.

Zimmerman, J. E., S. M. Shortell, W. A. Knaus, D. M. Rousseau, D. P. Wagner, R. R. Gillies, E. A. Draper, and K. Devers. 1993. "Value and Cost of Teaching Hospitals: A Prospective, Multicenter, Inception Cohort Study." *Critical Care Medicine* 21: 1,432–42.

Chapter Six

What Does Medicare Spending Buy Us?

David M. Cutler

The need for major Medicare reform is clear. In an era of tight government, Medicare is one of the few programs that is rapidly expanding. Medicare costs are increasing at over twice the growth rate of the tax revenues that fund the program. As a result, the Medicare program will exceed the revenues available to pay for it by the end of the next decade. We need to reduce the growth rate of Medicare costs to put the program on a stable long-term financing basis.

Both Democrats and Republicans agree with those statements. Consider a typical statement from President Clinton:

> I said the Medicare Trust Fund is in trouble, we have to do something to lengthen its life, we have to do the responsible thing and keep it strong, and I proposed solutions to keep it strong . . . We've got to do what it takes to save Medicare.

Or from Senate Majority Leader Trent Lott:

> Medicare is at risk because its spending is growing at rates that cannot be sustained. Frankly speaking, unless the necessary steps are taken to limit the rate of growth and preserve Medicare, it will be unable to pay for hospital care. . . . We must continue our efforts to preserve and protect Medicare, both for this generation and the next.

David M. Cutler is professor of economics at Harvard University and research associate at the National Bureau of Economic Research.

This paper was prepared for the conference Medicare Reform: Issues and Answers, held at Texas A&M University, 3 April 1998. I am grateful to the National Institutes on Aging for research support.

The two parties do not agree on how to reform Medicare, but they do agree it needs to spend less.

But how certain is the need for Medicare reform? And by how much should costs be cut? The *costs* of Medicare are certainly great. But costs are only half the issue. Medicare policy must also look at the *benefits* of the program. If the benefits of Medicare are greater than the costs, Medicare may be worth expanding, even if this means increasing taxes to pay for it.

Consider an analogy. Computer spending is much greater now than it used to be. Today, computer sales account for many billions of dollars, where they were virtually nonexistent fifty years ago. Is computer spending too high? Do we need national computer reform? The answer is clearly no. Computer spending is very valuable; computers add to productivity and make life easier. The same reasoning should apply to Medicare. Medicare costs should be reduced if the money spent on Medicare does not yield high returns. But Medicare should be unchanged, or even increased, if the spending is buying valuable services.[1]

The important question for policy, therefore, is how valuable is Medicare spending? The answer to this is not immediately clear. Consider two questions:

- Do you believe that Medicare operates (*a*) very efficiently or (*b*) relatively inefficiently?
- As a taxpayer and future Medicare beneficiary, would you rather have (*a*) the Medicare system that is currently available at its current cost or (*b*) the Medicare system as it existed in 1970 (including only 1970 medical technology) at its 1970 cost?

Informal surveys of these questions suggest that the vast majority of people answer (*b*) and (*a*)—people believe Medicare is very inefficient, but at the same time they like the increased services that Medicare has been able to provide, even at its higher cost. How can both of these statements be true? If Medicare is inefficient, why do people like it so much? If the program has brought so much value, why do people uniformly believe it should be smaller? Answering these questions is the key to successful Medicare reform.

In this chapter, I argue that people's answers to both questions are right, and they are not at all incompatible. On the whole, Medicare has been extremely valuable. Plausible estimates suggest that the return to Medicare spending in terms of better health has been higher than

Medicare costs—that it is good for society that Medicare has grown so rapidly. But this does not mean that all of Medicare services are valuable. Medicare has not developed mechanisms to limit the services it provides to those who will benefit from them greatly; as a result, Medicare pays for a lot of inefficient care.

It is the excessive utilization of services, and not the overall level of Medicare spending, that should drive the policy debate. Cost increases for valuable medical services are good for society, even if they require increased taxes to pay for them. But spending more on Medicare than is necessary is wasteful.

Focusing on the excessive utilization of services rather than overall Medicare costs leads me to four conclusions about Medicare reform. First, we should not put a budget on Medicare. Since the problem with Medicare is not the level of spending as a whole, budgeting the program as a whole does not make sense. Second, current mechanisms to reduce Medicare costs, which largely focus on reducing payments to providers, are not a good long-run system. Over time, the growth of Medicare spending has been predominantly a result of increased quantities of care being provided. Reducing prices cannot offset increases in the quantity of care over time. Third, moving some of the costs of Medicare from the government to the elderly is a good idea but cannot be the entire Medicare solution. Shifting costs from the government to the elderly is just that—a shift of the existing burden. It does not reduce the amount of overused services. Finally, a choice-based system for Medicare holds the most promise for limiting the use of inappropriate care. By giving beneficiaries a choice over insurance plans and making them pay more for more generous care, market forces can be used to direct care to its most valuable uses. The choice-based system is not easy to implement, but it is likely to be the most viable long-term proposal for Medicare reform.

I. The Cost of Medicare

I begin with basic data on the cost of Medicare. Medicare costs are substantial. Figure 6.1 shows real Medicare spending per beneficiary (in 1996 dollars), and table 6.1 shows decadal growth rates. The growth of Medicare is impressive. In 1970 Medicare spent about $1,400 per beneficiary. Over the next quarter century, spending increased by over 5 per-

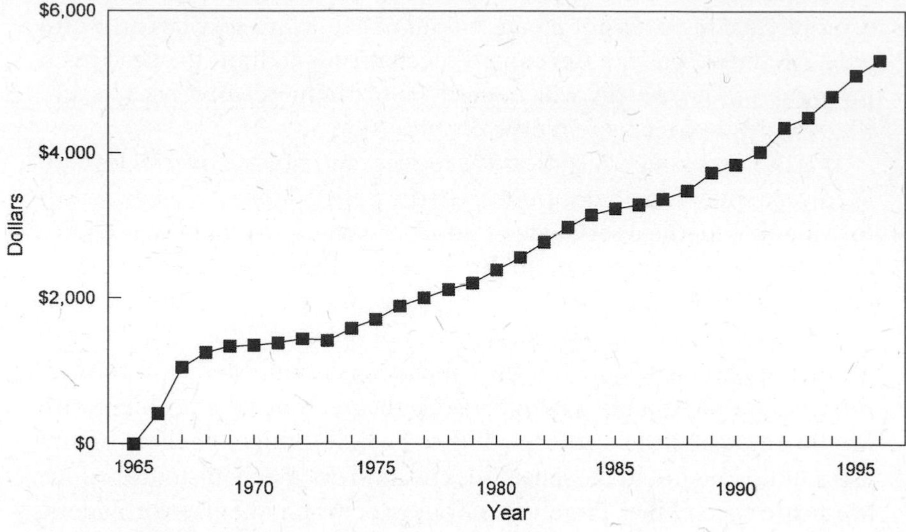

Figure 6.1 Medicare Spending per Beneficiary
Note: Spending is in 1996 dollars.

cent per year, to nearly $5,400 per beneficiary in 1996. To put this in perspective, the average person turning age 65 in 1994 (with a life expectancy around seventeen years) can expect to consume over $65,000 in Medicare services in their remaining life, even if Medicare spending at any age were constant for the rest of their life.

Of course, the increase in spending is not unique to Medicare. The second column of table 6.1 shows growth rates of non-Medicare spending. Between 1970 and 1990, the growth of non-Medicare costs was roughly equal to the growth of Medicare costs. Since 1990 non-Medicare costs have increased much less rapidly than Medicare costs.

Table 6.1 Growth of Medical Spending

Period	Medicare	Non-Medicare
1970–1996	5.3%	4.2%
1970–1980	5.7%	4.5%
1980–1990	4.7%	5.2%
1990–1996	5.4%	2.3%

NOTE: Growth rates are real, per person, and are annualized.

The commonality of cost growth between the public and private sectors over long periods of time suggests that there is no magic bullet for Medicare—that simply moving the system to the private sector would not necessarily reduce the growth of Medicare spending. Thus, it is important to think more deeply about potential Medicare reforms.

The key question in evaluating Medicare spending is to determine why Medicare costs have increased so rapidly. Is the Medicare cost increase a result of rising prices for medical services or a result of increasing quantities of services being provided? These two explanations have very different implications for Medicare reform. Increasing prices of services suggests a simple solution—administratively reduce prices and limit their growth rate. Cost increases driven by quantity increases, in contrast, present much more difficult policy problems, since this requires valuing the additional services provided.

Empirical research is virtually uniform in the conclusion that *the dominant factor in the growth of medical care costs over time is the increasing quantity of services provided, not increases in the price of given services.* I illustrate this finding with an example.[2] Consider the treatment of heart attacks: Heart attacks are expensive but not unusually technologically intensive, and their acute nature makes it easy to measure changes in treatment. There are about 230,000 new cases in the Medicare population annually,[3] making them a large share of Medicare's budget. In 1984 Medicare spent $2.6 billion on hospital care in the year following a heart attack (adjusted to 1991 dollars). This increased to $3.4 billion in 1991,[4] for an annual growth rate of 3.9 percent. The increasing cost of heart attack care is shown in the first row of table 6.2.

What accounts for this nearly 4 percent annual growth in spending on heart attacks? One potential explanation is an increase in the number of people with heart attacks. In fact, however, the number of new heart attacks was essentially constant from 1984 to 1991 (the second row of table 6.2). In contrast, spending per heart attack, shown in the third row of the table, increased by 4 percent annually between 1984 and 1991.

To understand what is responsible for cost growth, it helps to know more about the treatment of a heart attack. The least invasive treatment for heart attacks is medical management. This typically involves drug therapy (including clot-dissolving drugs), monitoring, and counseling and treatment for reducing risk factors such as high cholesterol

Table 6.2 Accounting for the Growth of Spending on Heart Attacks, 1984–91

AMI Treatment	Intensive Procedure Use			Average Reimbursement		
	1984	1991	Annual Change*	1984	1991	Annual Change
Total Spending				$2.6 bn	$3.4 bn	3.9%
Number of Patients				233,295	227,182	−0.4
Average Spending				$11,175	$14,772	4.0
Type of Treatment						
Medical Management	88.7%	59.4%	−4.2%	$9,829	$10,783	1.3%
Catheterization Only**	5.5	15.5	1.4	15,380	13,716	−1.6
Angioplasty	0.9	12.0	1.6	25,841	17,040	−5.9
Bypass Surgery	4.9	13.0	1.2	28,135	32,117	1.9

NOTE: Reimbursement for 1984 is in 1991 dollars, adjusted using the GDP deflator. Price and quantity indices use 1991 weights.

*Growth is average percentage point change each year.

**Patients who received catheterization but no revascularization procedure. Patients who received bypass surgery or angioplasty will also have had a catheterization.

levels and smoking. An alternative to medical management of a heart attack is to use one or more invasive cardiac procedures. Invasive treatment begins with a cardiac catheterization, a diagnostic procedure that documents areas of no or limited blood flow that may be involved in the current or possible subsequent heart attacks. If the catheterization detects important blockages in the arteries supplying the heart, more intensive revascularization procedures may be used to treat the blockages: coronary artery bypass surgery (CABG), a highly intensive open-heart surgical procedure to bypass occluded regions of the heart's blood flow; or percutaneous transluminal coronary angioplasty (PTCA), a procedure where a balloon-tipped catheter is inserted into the blocked artery and inflated with the goal of restoring blood flow.

Naturally, Medicare pays much more for patients receiving intensive surgery than for patients not receiving intensive surgery. As table 6.2 shows, in 1991 bypass surgery was reimbursed at three times the rate of medical management, and angioplasty was reimbursed 60 percent more than medical management. But these payments have not increased substantially over time. Payments for angioplasty, for example, fell as Medicare officials realized it was reimbursed too highly in 1984 relative to its true severity. Prices for the other services changed little in real terms.

Table 6.3 Accounting for the Growth of Heart Attack Spending

Component	**Share**
Total	100%
Quantity Increase	76%
Price Increase	6
Covariance	31

NOTE: Based on table 6.2.

In contrast, procedures use has increased substantially. As table 6.2 shows, in 1984, 11 percent of patients received a catheterization, with 5 percent of patients going on to receive bypass surgery and 1 percent receiving angioplasty. By 1991, 41 percent of patients received a catheterization, with 13 percent also receiving bypass surgery and 12 percent also receiving angioplasty.

How much of the rise in costs is because of this explosion in the use of high-tech procedures and how much is due to price changes? Table 6.3 shows the answer. Essentially all of the increase in spending is a result of increases in the quantity of intensive treatments provided. Price changes have had virtually no effect on increases in total spending.

The importance of quantity changes, and not price changes, in explaining the growth of Medicare costs has fundamental implications for Medicare reform. Most importantly, it means there are no easy solutions to Medicare costs. If Medicare spending is to be limited over the long term, it will necessarily mean that Medicare beneficiaries will receive fewer services. Of course, receiving fewer services is not bad if those services have little medical value. If the services have high value, however, reducing spending could have deleterious effects on the health of Medicare beneficiaries. This analysis thus highlights the fundamental importance of determining the value of medical services to the elderly.

II. The Benefits of Medicare

Traditional discussions of Medicare benefits have highlighted the increased access to medical providers that Medicare has allowed (Davis and Shoen 1978). Changes in access to medical care for the elderly have been impressive. Physicians visits, hospitalizations, and use of medical services all rose with the implementation of Medicare and have continued to increase since then. It is not difficult to understand why these changes occurred. Prior to the enactment of Medicare, only about half of the elderly had any insurance coverage. When people retired, they often lost their insurance coverage. And even the coverage the elderly had was not very generous (McClellan and Skinner 1997). Many insurance policies paid a fixed amount for a hospital stay (for example, $5 or $10 per day) excluding coverage for physician visits or prescription drugs.

But increasing medical *inputs* is not the ultimate goal of Medicare. The more important question is whether Medicare improved the *health* of the elderly. If the additional medical services were not sufficiently valuable, increased service provision would not have been worth the cost.

This analysis is a *social* cost-benefit calculation for the Medicare system. There are other questions that might also be asked about the *distribution* of the costs and benefits. For example, society may decide that it is worth it to provide additional Medicare services but may not want to place such a high burden of paying for that care on the nonelderly population. As in all economics, separating efficiency and distribution is critical. I focus on the efficiency issue of Medicare financing, leaving aside the distribution of the costs and benefits.

Commensurate with the birth of Medicare and its subsequent growth has been increased survival for the elderly. Figure 6.2 shows life expectancy for men and women conditional on reaching age 65.[5] Women reaching age 65 in 1990 could expect to live nearly 19 years, roughly 7 years more than women reaching age 65 at the turn of the century. For men, the improvement has been nearly 3-1/2 years. What is important about this figure is that most of the increase in life expectancy has occurred in the past few decades. Between 1900 and 1940, life expectancy at age 65 increased by only 1.4 years for women and 0.6 years for men. In the next two decades, life expectancy increased by 1 to 3 years. And since Medicare was passed, life expectancy at age 65 has increased by another 2 to 3 years.

The improvement in longevity since 1960 is fundamentally different from the improvement in the two preceding decades. Mortality reductions at mid-century were a result of the discovery of antibiotics. In 1940 death from infections and pneumonia were high; by 1960 they

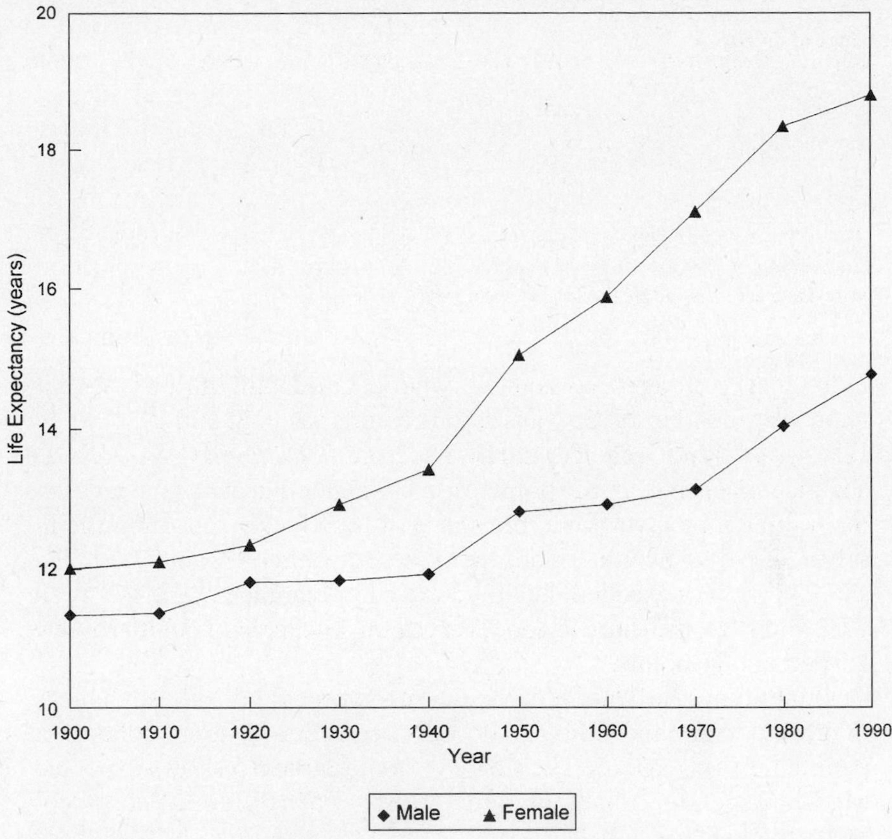

Figure 6.2 Life Expectancy at Age 65

were much lower. Mortality among the elderly was increasingly dominated by the chronic conditions of old age—cardiovascular disease and cancer in particular. Since the late 1960s, cardiovascular disease mortality has fallen by 3 percent annually. This reduction in cardiovascular disease mortality is the primary factor behind improved health for the elderly. Medicare almost certainly played an important role in the reduction in cardiovascular disease mortality.

Coupled with the reduction in mortality has been an increase in health among those who are alive. Table 6.4 shows changes in the self-reported health of the elderly over time. The Health Interview Survey asks people: "How would you rate your health as compared with other

Table 6.4 Self-Reported Health Status of the Elderly

Share of Elderly Reporting Health As:	1972	1981	1982	1994
Excellent	30.1%	28.6%	14.9%	15.8%
Very Good		—	19.1	23.0
Good	38.1	40.7	30.4	33.1
Fair	22.4	21.5	22.8	18.1
Poor	8.5	8.6	11.7	9.4

NOTE: Data are from the Health Interview Survey.

individuals your age: excellent, very good, good, fair, or poor?"[6] *Very good* was added in 1982; I thus report results for 1972 and 1981, when *very good* was not a choice, and for 1982 and 1994, when *very good* was a choice. In each year, the population is weighted using a constant demographic mix. Over time, the share of the elderly reporting themselves in better health conditions rose. Between 1972 and 1981, the share in good or excellent health rose by 1 percentage point. Between 1982 and 1994, the share in good, very good, or excellent health rose by 7.5 percentage points.

Quantifying the benefits of Medicare requires valuing these changes in morbidity and mortality. To do this, I consider different cohorts of people reaching age 65. The first column of table 6.5 shows expected Medicare spending for people who reach age 65 in different years. People reaching age 65 in 1970 could expect to spend nearly $14,000 of

Table 6.5 Expected Medicare Spending and Health for New Medicare Eligibles

	Spending		Value of Life		
Year Reaching Age 65	Medicare Spending	Change in Spending	Length of Life	Quality of Life	Change in QALYs
1970	$13,723	—	15.2	.30	—
1980	28,334	$14,612	16.4	.33	$85,200
1990	50,089	21,754	16.7	.37	76,700
1994	67,702	17,614	17.4	.39	53,740
Change	—	$53,980	—	—	$215,640

NOTE: Spending data are for 1967, 1977, and 1987. Quality of life is from Cutler and Richardson (1997). Value of a quality-adjusted life-year is assumed to be $100,000.

Medicare resources over their remaining lifetime, while people who reached age 65 in 1994 could expect to spend nearly $70,000 in Medicare resources over their remaining lifetime, for an increase of over $50,000 per person (the second column of the table).

Valuing the health of the elderly is more difficult, since it requires estimating the worth of life itself. To estimate the value of health, I use the concept of "Quality Adjusted Life-Years" (QALYs). I assume that a person's health in every year of life can be scaled on a 0 to 1 basis, where 0 is death and 1 is perfect health. Living with particular conditions falls between 0 and 1. For example, people who have had a stroke will have lower quality of life than those who have not had a stroke—their ability to walk or take part in everyday activities may be impaired; they may be in a nursing home; they may be depressed; and so on. Thus, health for a stroke survivor will be lower than health for a person who has not had a stroke.

Measuring these quality-of-life factors for people who have suffered a stroke or any other serious condition is very difficult. In work I have done elsewhere (Cutler and Richardson 1997, 1998), I have estimated quality-of-life weights for a number of common conditions and examined how those weights changed over time. The procedure involved is relatively simple: I use survey data like that reported above to compare the self-reported health of people with and without certain conditions. For example, people who have survived a major cardiovascular incident generally report themselves in worse health than people who have not suffered such an illness. I then scale these self-reported health measures within the 0 to 1 interval. The result is a set of health weights for different conditions. For example, having survived a serious cardiovascular disease incident reduces quality of life by 30 to 40 percent; minor hearing problems reduce quality of life by only 5 to 10 percent. Table 6.5 shows the resulting estimates of quality of life. The third column shows life expectancy conditional on reaching age 65. Life expectancy increased 2.2 years between 1970 and 1994. The fourth column shows the quality-of-life weights. Quality of life was about 0.3 in 1970, and increased to approximately 0.4 by 1990. The generally low level of quality of life reflects the accumulated effects of aging and the high prevalence rate of adverse conditions in the elderly (such as arthritis, vision problems, and hearing problems). The increase in quality of life over time reflects an improvement in physical and mental functioning for the elderly with these conditions. Over the time period Medicare has been in place, quality of life for people with a wide range of conditions has improved by 5 to 10 percent.

Multiplying the expected number of life-years remaining by the quality of life in those years yields the expected number of quality-adjusted life-years for the average person reaching age 65. To compare this to medical spending, we need to value these life-years in dollars. Estimating the value of a year of life is quite difficult. Some estimates of the value of life look only at the net contribution of people: what people earn less what they consume. It is generally accepted that this is a poor way to measure the value of life, however. The elderly, for example, would have negative value for society, since they consume more than they produce. Instead, most people accept that there is an intrinsic "value of being alive" that a person, and thus society, has. For example, people have estimated this intrinsic value in several ways. People have to be paid more to work in risky occupations than in safer occupations, to offset the increased hazards. Using information on the risks in different jobs and how much more people have to be paid to work in those jobs yields an estimate of how much people value their life. In other settings, people purchase safety devices, such as airbags and fire alarms. The amount that people are willing to pay for these goods is a second way to estimate people's underlying value of a life. A survey of estimates in the literature suggests a dollar value of a year of life of approximately \$75,000 to \$150,000 (Tolley et al. 1994; Viscusi 1993). As a consensus estimate, I assume a year of life is worth \$100,000.

The last column of table 6.5 shows the change in the dollar value of quality-adjusted life-years over time. In the past quarter century, health of the elderly has improved by about \$215,000. The \$215,000 increase in the value of life is greater than the \$50,000 increase in Medicare spending; indeed, this is true for every decade over this time period. Thus, if all of the improvement in health were a result of increased Medicare spending, the spending on Medicare would clearly be worth the money.

Of course, many factors other than Medicare account for improved health—reduced smoking, better exercise, and less physical stress during working years. Still, even if only one-quarter of the improvement in health were a result of increased Medicare spending, the additional spending on Medicare would be worth it. While there is no definitive calculation about how much of the improvement in health results from Medicare, I suspect the share is over one-quarter.[7] Thus, the calculations suggest that increased Medicare spending is worth its cost.

Table 6.6 The Net Benefits of Heart Attack Treatment

	Spending		Value of Life	
Year	**Costs**	**Change in Costs**	**Life Expectancy**	**Change in Life Value**
1984	$11,123	—	5-2/12	—
1985	11,638	$514	5-4/12	$11,282
1986	11,980	856	5-4/12	13,108
1987	12,250	1,127	5-5/12	20,721
1988	12,746	1,622	5-6/12	31,196
1989	13,076	1,953	5-8/12	43,557
1990	13,681	2,558	5-9/12	54,547
1991	14,851	3,727	5-10/12	59,442

NOTE: The sample is all elderly Medicare beneficiaries with a new heart attack. Costs are in 1991 dollars.

An Example: The Costs and Benefits of Heart Attack Treatment

To provide further evidence on the conclusions noted above, I use the example of treatment of heart attacks. Table 6.6 shows calculations of the costs and benefits of heart attack care. The first two columns of the table show heart attack costs. Between 1984 and 1991, heart attack costs increased by nearly $4,000 in real terms, as noted in table 6.6.[8]

There have also been improvements in health outcomes for heart attack patients. Figure 6.3 shows cumulative mortality rates for the elderly at various time periods after a heart attack: 1 day; 90 days; and 1 through 5 years. Mortality after a heart attack has decreased dramatically over time.[9] The third column of table 6.6 shows the change in life expectancy implied by these mortality reductions. In 1984 the average person with a heart attack lived 5 years and 2 months. By 1991 the average heart attack sufferer lived 5 years and 10 months, an increase of 8 months. There might also have been morbidity changes after a heart attack. Data on this are difficult to compile, however; few studies have evaluated the detailed functional capabilities (Can people walk up a flight of stairs without pain?) of people with a heart attack over time. I thus consider only the mortality benefits of changes in heart attack therapies.

Assuming that a year of life is again worth $100,000, the last column of table 6.6 shows the change in the value of life after a heart attack. Be-

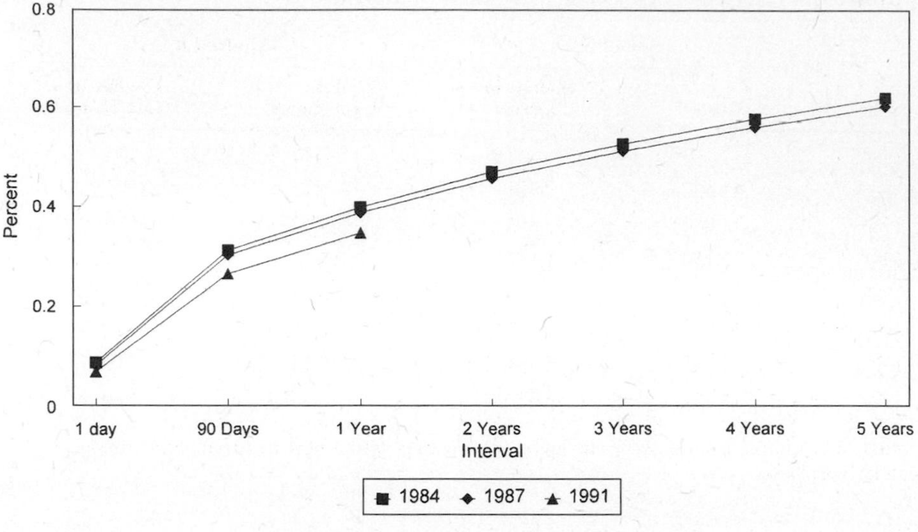

Figure 6.3 Mortality after a Heart Attack

tween 1984 and 1991, the value of additional life increased by nearly $60,000. Comparing the second and fourth columns of table 6.6 shows a clear result—the value of additional life is substantially in excess of the increase in costs of heart attack care. Indeed, the improvement in health would be greater than its cost even if only one-quarter of the mortality reductions were a result of Medicare spending. Thus, looking at care for a particular condition leads to very similar results as the aggregate analysis: *Taken as a whole, the increase in Medicare spending over time has almost certainly yielded health improvements greater than Medicare's cost.*

III. Is All of Medicare Worth It?

While Medicare spending as a whole is likely worth its cost, there is other data showing that *a substantial amount of Medicare spending buys little in the way of health benefits*. Perhaps the most widely noted evidence for this view comes from detailed analysis of the appropriateness of particular medical procedures. A series of studies have examined how appropriate medical care is in common clinical settings. The studies usually begin by specifying guidelines for appropriate and inappropriate treatment. These guidelines, developed with physician input, detail the conditions under which a given medical procedure is appropriate and the conditions under which it is inappropriate. Researchers then gather data on actual treatments and examine how frequently procedures that are applied are performed appropriately or inappropriately.

Figure 6.4 shows the results of some of these studies. As much as one-third of medical care provided is clearly inappropriate or of equivocal value. This is true for a wide range of very common conditions. Further, these studies might understate the amount of inappropriate medical care. Appropriate medical care in these studies is defined as any care whose expected benefit is greater than the risk involved to the patient. The cost of the care being provided is not considered. From society's perspective, appropriate medical care is care that has benefits greater than the risks involved to the patient *plus* the cost of that care to society, since resources spent providing medical care to the sick are resources that are not consumed elsewhere. At least some of the care that these studies judge to be appropriate would likely have costs greater

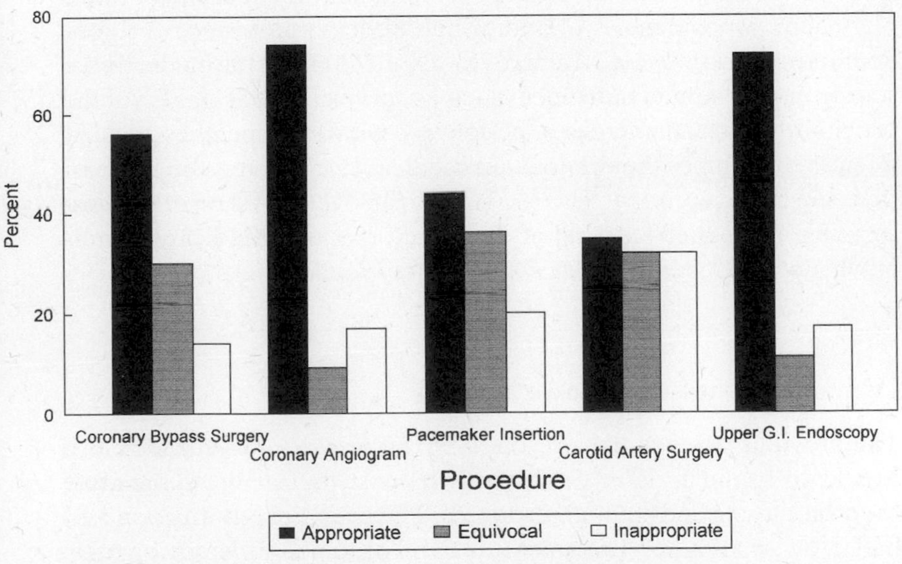

Figure 6.4 Inappropriate Care for Common Procedures
SOURCE: The Rand Corporation

than expected health benefits and would therefore be inappropriate from society's perspective.[10]

In addition to this type of study, there is a great deal of other evidence that some medical care has little or no value. For example, the Rand Health Insurance Experiment (Newhouse et al. 1993) found that people who were better insured used more medical care than those who had less generous insurance, but that health outcomes were no different. Other research shows that differences in the use of medical care in different areas of the country (Wennberg et al. 1987), in different hospitals (Staiger and Gaumer 1990; Cutler 1995), or over time (Garber, Fuchs, and Silverman 1984; Kahn et al. 1990; Cutler and Staiger 1996) frequently keep people alive for several months but not as long as a year.

These finding are not surprising in light of the incentives built into the Medicare system, and the medical care system more generally. Medicare beneficiaries pay little for medical care at the time they receive services. Thus, beneficiaries have incentives to demand care with any value, even if that value is low. Coupled with this demand side effect are problems from incomplete information. Patients cannot always tell what services they should receive. As a result, people frequently make decisions on the recommendation of doctors. Since physicians are paid more for additional services performed, however, doctors have incentives to overprovide care. Finally, in the medical care setting, highly valued outcomes (such as survival) are at stake. As the probability of death increases, people are willing to spend essentially all of the resources they control on medical care, even if the value of that care to society is low. This too leads to an overprovision of medical services. The net effect of all of these factors is that Medicare spends much more on medical services than society would like.

IV. Implications for Medicare Reform

The previous two sections present a mixed message about Medicare. Medicare spending is in total worth its cost, but at the same time Medicare wastes substantial resources. The program is both good and bad. How can this be? The answer is familiar to people watching their weight who sneak an extra diet milkshake: one can have too much of a good thing. Medicare as a whole has been extremely valuable—it has brought benefits far in excess of its costs. But we have overindulged. Many people receive services when society would be better off if they did not. The problem with Medicare is not so much that spending is so high, but that Medicare has no mechanism to allocate care where it is appropriate and deny care where it is inappropriate. As a result, treatments are frequently provided both to people who really benefit from them and people who will benefit only a little.

As a public policy matter, the unfortunate conclusion is that we are asking the wrong question. The question that is frequently posed in the policy context is *How can we contain the costs of Medicare so that we can afford it in the current government budget?* That question, however, misses the point. Instead, we should be asking a different question: *How can we preserve the components of costs that are beneficial but limit care when it is inappropriate*? This may fit Medicare into the current budget, or it may not. But we will never get the right answer to Medicare's problems if we do not ask the right questions.

Answering this other question fully is beyond the scope of this chapter (see Cutler 1996 for more discussion). Some conclusions flow naturally from this analysis, however.

Implication 1: Putting a Budget on Medicare Is a Poor Idea

Budget caps are valuable when we know how much we want to spend and the issue is how to enforce that amount. But in Medicare, we do not know how much we want to spend. While we can guess the amount of inappropriate care, we do not know it for certain. And even if we knew it for certain, there is no guarantee that the care that would be eliminated if a cap were in place is the care that is of low value. More fundamentally, budget caps do not create incentives to provide medical care more efficiently. Thus, they do not address the underlying Medicare problem.

Implication 2: The Methods for Containing Medicare Costs That the Government Has Used in the Past Are Not a Long-Term Solution

Traditional cost containment methods in Medicare have focused on reducing the prices paid to providers. For example, in the recent Balanced Budget Act, most of the Medicare savings come from reducing the payment rates to hospitals and physicians. The major reason why

Medicare costs are increasing, however, is because the *quantity* of services provided is rising, not because the *price* of services is rising. Focusing on cutting prices will be ineffective when the underlying source of Medicare cost increases is increasing quantities of care.

Implication 3: Making the Elderly Pay More for Medicare Is a Good Policy but Cannot Be the Entire Solution

A common set of reform proposals is to increase the cost of Medicare to beneficiaries. There are many ways to do this—raising the Part B premium, having people save for Medicare during their working years, means-testing eligibility, and so on. These proposals would effectively transfer some of the costs of Medicare from the public sector to the private sector.

Many of these proposals have merit. When the elderly are as well-off as they are and many of the nonelderly are as poor as they are, it makes sense to transfer some of the Medicare burden from the nonelderly to the elderly. But as with the emphasis on price cutting, these proposals do not address the issue of excessive Medicare services. Transferring costs from the nonelderly to the elderly merely shifts the overall burden of the program; it does not eliminate wasteful care. To address the issue of wasteful care, reforms need to change the incentives to overprovide these services.

Implication 4: Restructuring the Medicare System into a Choice-based System Could Facilitate the Necessary Reduction in Inappropriate Services

Ultimately, there are two ways to limit medical care to those who benefit from it most: make individuals pay more for the services they receive at the time they receive them (reducing demand for care) or provide incentives for providers to supply less care (reducing supply of care). Moving in the first of these directions would require increasing the cost sharing in Medicare. Medicare out-of-pocket payments, for example, would have to increase, and Medigap policies would be prohibited from covering these costs. Moving in the second of these directions is the goal of "managed care" insurance.

Private insurance policies used to be very similar to the current Medicare policy. People chose whichever provider they wanted, and they faced only a small out-of-pocket cost for doing so. In the private sector, however, that type of plan has essentially been eliminated. In its place, medical care is now managed—patients need approval from a physician to receive particular services; they are limited in which providers they can see; providers are subject to review for what they do; and providers are given financial incentives to provide less care. The potential gain from managed care is its ability to induce providers to eliminate wasteful care. If plans can do this, they can attract more enrollees and make a profit.

Market forces might be harnessed to meet these goals in Medicare as well. A reformed Medicare system would probably look like most employer health programs today: the employer offers a menu of policy choices and contributes a fixed amount for health insurance. Employees take that contribution and pay the additional amount (if any) for the plan they want. Generous, and thus high-cost, plans will be those with less cost sharing on the part of the employee and less management of care. Employees who want a particularly generous plan will pay more than those who want a less generous plan. Thus, employees will be encouraged to choose higher cost-sharing plans or more managed care plans if the additional cost of more generous insurance is not worth its benefits. In such an environment, plans would compete to be low cost. Low-cost plans will attract more enrollees, assuming the cost reduction does not result from limiting access to very valuable care. Plans that are inefficient will not attract enrollees.

If that is the goal, however, the reality is quite complicated. A competitive model for Medicare is *not* the same as a competitive model for other industries (see, for example, Cutler and Reber 1998 and Cutler and Zeckhauser 1998). Consider just a few of the difficulties. Competition requires that individuals be informed about the options facing them and the value of different choices; in medical care such information is far from perfect. Indeed, the lack of good information about appropriate medical care has provoked enormous public concern. The strong public reaction against managed care insurers, I believe, is directly related to the lack of information people have about how medical decisions are made. When people do not know what is appropriate care, they fear that for-profit insurers will deny them valuable treatment just to save a few dollars. If people were more aware of what care was available and appropriate for them, there might be much less concern about insurers limiting utilization.

Competition also requires that sick people not have to pay more for health insurance or be turned away simply because they are sick. In a laissez-faire insurance market, both of these will happen. Insurers will not want to insure people they know to be sick, or they will charge them very high prices. Preventing this will require substantial regulation. Insurers will have to accept everyone who applies; they will have to renew everyone who wants renewal; prices will not be allowed to vary across individuals. And the government will need to compensate plans that differentially attract sick people instead of healthy people. A generous plan, for example, will be populated more by the sick than the healthy. As a result, it will have very high premiums, owing solely to who enrolls in the plan, not the plan's true generosity. These high premiums will discourage both sick and healthy from enrolling in these plans, even if these people were willing to pay the additional costs they personally would use in the more generous plan. This phenomenon is termed adverse selection, and it is a very important danger. The government will need to limit adverse selection, most likely by providing indirect subsidies to the most generous plans (Newhouse 1996).

Market-based Medicare reform is not without risk. But it is perhaps the only option on the table that addresses the underlying problems in the Medicare program. Designing a workable system of marketplace incentives into Medicare is perhaps the most pressing issue in Medicare reform.

Notes

1. One might argue that the difference between Medicare and computers is that the government pays for Medicare but not for computers. This is not true, however. The federal government purchases computers directly and also subsidizes them indirectly, through the tax deduction for business purchases of equipment.

2. The example is taken from Cutler and McClellan (1996) and Cutler, McClellan, Newhouse, and Remler (1998).

3. These figures exclude the elderly enrolled in managed care. This is a growing, but small, share of the elderly population.

4. Total Medicare spending on inpatient care was $63 billion in 1991.

5. The estimates are from period life tables; they use age-specific mortality in any year to forecast life expectancy for people alive at that time.

6. *Very good* was not included as an option until the mid-1980s.

7. One might be tempted to extrapolate health improvements from the pre-

Medicare period to determine what would have happened if Medicare had not been created. But the source of health improvements differs so much over time that this seems problematic. For example, health improvements in the 1940–1960 period were largely the result of the development of penicillin and other antibiotics. Since 1960, in contrast, reductions in cardiovascular disease mortality have been the most important source of mortality reductions. While it may be that this change would have occurred even in the absence of Medicare, it is not obvious that this is the case.

8. Cost data differ slightly from table 6.2 because this table holds constant the demographic mix of the population.

9. Because the mortality data only extend through the end of 1992, mortality rates in 1991 cannot be measured for time periods longer than one year.

10. On the other side, some have claimed that the studies overstate the amount of inappropriate care by classifying some appropriate care as inappropriate.

References

Chassin, Mark, et al. 1987. "Does Inappropriate Use Explain Geographic Variations in the Use of Health Care Services?" *Journal of the American Medical Association* 258: 2,533–37.

Cutler, David M. 1995. "The Incidence of Adverse Medical Outcomes under Prospective Payment." *Econometrica* (February): 29–50.

———. 1996. "Restructuring Medicare for the Future." In *Setting National Priorities*, edited by R. Reischauer. Washington, D.C.: Brookings Institution.

Cutler, David M., and Mark McClellan. 1996. "The Determinants of Technological Change in Heart Attack Treatment," mimeo.

Cutler, David M., Mark McClellan, Joseph P. Newhouse, and Dahlia Remler. 1998. "Are Medical Prices Declining?" *Quarterly Journal of Economics* (November): 991–1,024.

Cutler, David M., and Sarah J. Reber. 1998. "Paying for Health Insurance: The Tradeoff between Competition and Adverse Selection." *Quarterly Journal of Economics* (May): 433–66.

Cutler, David M., and Elizabeth Richardson. 1997. "Measuring the Health of the United States Population." *Brookings Papers on Economic Activity: Microeconomics*. Washington, D.C.: Brookings Institution, pp. 217–71.

———. 1998. "The Value of Health, 1970–1990." *American Economic Review* (May): 97–100.

Cutler, David M., and Douglas Staiger. 1996. "Measuring the Benefits of Medical Progress," mimeo. Harvard University.

Cutler, David M., and Richard J. Zeckhauser 1998. "Adverse Selection in Health Insurance." In *Frontiers in Health Economics*, edited by A. Garber. Cambridge: MIT Press.

Davis, Karen, and Cathy Schoen. 1978. *Health and the War on Poverty: A Ten-Year Appraisal*. Washington, D.C.: Brookings Institution.

Garber, Alan, Victor Fuchs, and James Silverman. 1984. "Case Mix, Costs and Outcomes." *New England Journal of Medicine* (10 May): 1,231–37.

Greenspan, Allan M., et al. 1988. "Incidence of Unwarranted Implantation of Permanent Cardiac Pacemakers in a Large Medical Population." *New England Journal of Medicine* 318: 158–63.

Kahn, Katherine L., et al. 1990. "Comparing Outcomes of Care before and after Implementation of the DRG-Based Prospective Payment System." *Journal of the American Medical Association* 264 (15): 1,984–88.

McClellan, Mark, and Jonathan Skinner. 1997. "The Incidence of Medicare." NBER Working Paper No. 6013 (April).

Newhouse, Joseph P. 1993. *Free for All? Lessons from the Rand Health Insurance Experiment*. Cambridge: Harvard University Press.

———. 1996. "Reimbursing Health Plans and Health Providers: Selection versus Efficiency in Production." *Journal of Economic Literature* (September): 1,236–63.

Staiger, Doug, and Gary Gaumer. 1990. "The Effect of Prospective Payment on Post-Hospital Mortality." mimeo.

Tolley, George, Donald Kenkel, and Robert Fabian, eds. 1994. *Valuing Health for Policy: An Economic Approach*. Chicago: University of Chicago Press.

Viscusi, W. Kip. 1993. "The Value of Risks to Life and Health." *Journal of Economic Literature*, pp. 1,912–46.

Wennberg, Jack E., J. L. Freeman, and W. J. Culp. 1987. "Are Hospitals Services Rationed in New Haven or Over-Utilized in Boston?" *Lancet* 1 (23 May): 1,185–88.

Winslow, Constance M., et al. 1988a. "The Appropriateness of Carotid Endarterectomy." *New England Journal of Medicine* 318: 721–27.

Winslow, Constance M., et al. 1988b. "The Appropriateness of Performing Coronary Artery Bypass Surgery." *Journal of the American Medical Association* 260: 505–10.

Chapter Seven

Medicare from the Perspective of Generational Accounting

Jagadeesh Gokhale
Laurence J. Kotlikoff

I. Introduction

Notwithstanding all the attention being paid to our nation's current budget surplus, the U.S. fiscal position is grave. Unless policies are changed and changed soon, future American generations can expect to pay fifty cents of every dollar they earn to local, state, and federal governments in net taxes (taxes paid net of transfer payments received). This 50 percent lifetime net tax rate is roughly 70 percent larger than the rate current workers are slated to pay over their lifetimes.

This estimated imbalance in U.S. generational policy emerges from the latest U.S. generational accounting prepared by Gokhale, Page, and Sturrock (1999). Their study incorporates recent changes in fiscal policy, recent demographic projections, recent forecasts of government spending, and recent projections of expenditures on social insurance programs, including Social Security, Medicare, and Medicaid.

Although the current imbalance in U.S. generational policy is huge, it's much smaller than that estimated four years ago by Auerbach, Gokhale, and Kotlikoff (1995) and the Congressional Budget Office (1995). In those studies, the lifetime net tax rate confronting future gen-

Jagadeesh Gokhale is an economic adviser at the Federal Reserve Bank of Cleveland.
Laurence J. Kotlikoff is professor of economics at Boston University and a research associate of the National Bureau of Economic Research.

erations was roughly 80 percent. The dramatic reduction in the imbalance in generational policy reflects both changes in policies and revisions in projections of the amounts U.S. governments will receive and spend under existing policy.

Some of the revisions in the government's fiscal forecasts are quite remarkable. Take Medicare expenditures between 2030 and 2040. Compared with their 1995 projections, the Health Care Financing Administration (HCFA) is now projecting these expenditures to be 2 to 3 percentage points smaller. To put this revised projection in perspective, Medicare expenditures are now roughly 2.5 percent of GDP. Hence, the new HCFA forecast eliminates future Medicare expenditures in the 2030s, which, when measured relative to the size of the economy, are as large as the entire current Medicare program!

This chapter considers the role of Medicare in contributing to the imbalance in U.S. generational policy. It also describes the recent revisions in long-term Medicare expenditure projections, and it considers the extent to which immediate or future cuts in Medicare benefits can be used to eliminate the outstanding imbalance in U.S. generational policy. The chapter begins in the next section by reviewing the methodology of generational accounting. Section III presents baseline U.S. generational accounts, and section IV compares the imbalance in U.S. generational accounts with those in other developed countries. Section V describes the recent revision in projected Medicare expenditures and the ways balance can be restored to U.S. generational policy by cutting these expenditures.

II. The Method of Generational Accounting

This section draws heavily on Auerbach and Kotlikoff (1999) in summarizing the standard method of generational accounting. This methodology was first developed in Auerbach, Gokhale and Kotlikoff (1991).

Generational accounting is based on the government's intertemporal budget constraint, which is given in equation (1). This constraint requires that the remaining lifetime net tax payments of current generations and the lifetime net tax payments of future generations suffice, in present value, to cover the government's bills—the present value of its future spending on goods and services as well as its official net indebtedness. This constraint doesn't imply that the government ever retire its debt, only that it services at each point in time all debt that remains outstanding.

$$(1)\quad \sum_{k=t-D}^{t} N_{t,k} + (1+r)^{-(k-t)} \sum_{k=t+1}^{\infty} N_{t,k} = \sum_{s=t}^{\infty} G_s(1+r)^{-(s-t)} + D_t$$

The first term on the left side of (1) sums the *generational accounts*—the present value of the remaining lifetime net payments—of existing generations. The term $N_{t,k}$ stands for the account of the generation born in year k. The index k in this summation runs from $t-D$ (those age D, the maximum length of life, in year 0) to t (those born in year 0).

The second summation on the left side of (1) adds together the present values of the generational accounts of future generations, with k again representing the year of birth. To measure the value of these prospective future generational accounts as of time t, we need to discount these accounts to time t. We do so by using the economy's real before-tax rate of return, r.

The first term on the right-hand side of (1) expresses the present value of government consumption. In this summation, the values of government consumption in year s, given by G_s, are also discounted to year t. The remaining term on the right-hand side, D_t, denotes the government's net debt in year t—its explicit debt minus its assets, which consist of its financial assets plus the market value of state enterprises and extractable resources.

Equation (1) indicates the zero-sum nature of intergenerational fiscal policy. Holding the present value of government consumption fixed, a reduction in the present value of net taxes extracted from current generations (a decline in the first summation on the left side of [1]) necessitates an increase in the present value of net tax payments of future generations.

The generational account $N_{t,k}$ is defined by

$$(2)\qquad N_{t,k} = \sum_{s=\kappa}^{k+D} T_{s,k} P_{s,k} (1+r)^{-(s-\kappa)}$$

where $\kappa = \max(t,k)$. In expression (2), $T_{s,k}$ stands for the projected average net tax payment to the government made in year s by a member of the generation born in year k. The term $P_{s,k}$ stands for the number of surviving members of the cohort in year s who were born in year k. For generations born prior to year t, the summation begins in year t and all net taxes are discounted back to year t. For generations born in year $k > t$, the summation begins in year k and is discounted to that year.

A set of generational accounts is simply a set of values of $N_{t,k}$, one for each existing and future generation, with the property that the combined present value adds up to the right-hand side of equation (1). Though we distinguish male and female cohorts in many of the results presented below, we suppress sex subscripts in (1) and (2) to limit notation.

Note that generational accounts reflect only taxes paid less transfer payments received. With the exception of government expenditures on health care, which are treated as transfer payments, the accounts do not impute to particular generations the value of the government's purchases of goods and services because it is difficult to attribute the benefits of such purchases.[1] Therefore, the accounts do not show the full net benefit or burden that any generation receives from government policy as a whole, although they can show a generation's net benefit or burden from a particular policy change that affects only taxes and transfers. Thus, generational accounting tells us which generations will pay for government spending not included in the accounts, rather than telling us which generations will benefit from that spending. This implies nothing about the value of government spending; that is, there is no assumption, explicit or implicit, concerning the value to households of government purchases.

Assessing the Fiscal Burden Facing Future Generations

Given the right-hand side of equation (1) and the first term on the left-hand side of (1), we determine, as a residual, the value of the second term on the left-hand side of (1)—the collective payment, measured as a time t present value, required of future generations. Based on this amount, we determine the average present value lifetime net tax payment of each member of each future generation under the assumption that the average lifetime tax payment of successive generations rises at the economy's rate of productivity growth. This makes the lifetime payment a constant share of lifetime income. Controlling for this growth adjustment, the lifetime net tax payments of future generations are directly comparable with those of current newborns, since the generational accounts of both newborns and future generations take into account net tax payments over these generations' entire lifetimes and are discounted back to their respective years of birth.

Another way of measuring the imbalance of fiscal policy, illustrated below, is to ask what permanent change in some tax or transfer instrument—such as an immediate and permanent increase in income taxes or reduction in old-age Social Security benefits—would be necessary to equalize the lifetime growth-adjusted fiscal burden facing current newborns and future generations. Because such policies satisfy the government's intertemporal budget constraint, they are sustainable.

Generational Accounting versus Deficit Accounting

A final and critically important point to make about generational accounting is that the size of the fiscal burden confronting future generations (the second summation on the left-hand side of [1]), the generational accounts of newborn generations, and the imbalance in generational policy (measured as the difference in the accounts of newborns and the growth-adjusted accounts of future generations) are all invariant to the government's fiscal labeling—how it describes its receipts and payments.

The same, unfortunately, is not true of the government's official debt. As described in Kotlikoff (1992), from the perspective of neoclassical economic theory, neither the government's official debt nor its change over time—the deficit—is a well-defined economic concept. Rather these are accounting constructs whose values are entirely dependent on the choice of fiscal vocabulary. Stated differently, a government's reported debt and deficit bear no intrinsic relationship to any aspect of its fiscal policy, including its generational policy.

For example, if one calls past and future U.S. Social Security contributions "loans" to the government and past and future Social Security benefit payments "return of principal plus interest on these loans" less an "old-age net tax," the U.S. government's official debt becomes roughly $9 trillion larger than the "official" value. In terms of equation (1), this alternative but equally legitimate choice of language entails a higher value of the generational accounts of all existing generations, apart from newborns, as well as a higher value of official debt. The larger value of the debt term on the right-hand side of the equation is exactly matched by a higher value of the first summation on the left-hand side of the equation. Consequently, the size of the second summation on the left-hand side of the equation—the collective net tax burden facing future generations—is unchanged.

Each choice of fiscal language raises or lowers the first summation on the left-hand side of (1) and the official net debt term on the left-hand side by exactly the same amount. Because of the infinite ways to label each dollar given to the government by the private sector or given to the private sector by the government, there are infinite sets of alternative time series of the government's official debt that can be constructed simply by describing past and future economic policy with different words.[2] But none of these times series of debts and deficits, in and of themselves, tells us anything about how the government is treating alternative generations. Hence, generational accounting's message is not simply that we can do better than conventional deficit accounting in assessing the generational stance of fiscal policy, but also that deficit accounting—notwithstanding its routine use by every country in the world—is entirely devoid of economic content.

Assumptions Underlying Generational Account Calculations

To produce generational accounts, we require projections of population, taxes, transfers, and government expenditures; an initial value of government net debt; and a discount rate. We consider the impact of total, as opposed to just federal, government. Typically, we assume that government purchases grow at the same rate as GDP, although in some cases we break these purchases down into age-specific components and assume that each component remains constant per member of the relevant population, adjusted for the overall growth of GDP per capita. This causes different components of government purchases to grow more or less rapidly than GDP according to whether the relevant population grows or shrinks as a share of the overall population.

Government infrastructure purchases are treated like other forms of purchases in the calculations. Although such purchases provide an ongoing stream rather than a one-time amount of services, they must still be paid for. Generational accounting clarifies which generation or generations will have to bear the burden of these and other purchases. For government debt, we measure the government's net financial debt—its official debt less its official financial assets. We do not include the real assets of state enterprises in this measure, but instead subtract projected net profits from state enterprises from projected government spending. This procedure effectively capitalizes the value of these enterprises.

Government assets do not include the value of the government's existing infrastructure, such as parks. Including such assets would have no impact on the estimated fiscal burden facing future generations because including these assets would require adding to the projected flow of government purchases an offsetting flow of imputed rent on the government's existing infrastructure.

Aggregate taxes and transfer payments reported for the government sector in the National Income and Product Accounts are each broken down into several categories. Our general rule regarding tax incidence is to assume that taxes are borne by those paying the taxes, when the taxes are paid: income taxes on income, consumption taxes on consumers, and property taxes on property owners. There are two exceptions here, both of which involve capital income taxes. First, we distinguish between marginal and inframarginal capital income taxes. Inframarginal capital income taxes are distributed to existing wealth holders, whereas marginal capital income taxes are based on future projected wealth holdings. Second, in the case of small open economies, marginal corporate income taxes are assumed to be borne by (and are therefore allocated to) labor.

The typical method used to project the average values of particular taxes and transfer payments by age and sex starts with government forecasts of the aggregate amounts of each type of tax (for example, payroll) and transfer payment (for example, welfare benefits) in future years. These aggregate amounts are then distributed by age and sex based on cross-section-relative age-tax and age-transfer profiles derived from cross-section micro data sets. For years beyond those for which government forecasts are available, age- and sex-specific average tax and transfer amounts are assumed to equal those for the latest year for which forecasts are available, with an adjustment for growth.[3]

III. Baseline U.S. Generational Accounts

Tables 7.1 and 7.2 present baseline U.S. generational accounts for males and females. The base year for this analysis is 1995, but the fiscal

Table 7.1 U.S. Male Generational Accounts (present values in thousands of 1995 dollars, $r = .06, g = .012$)

Age in 1995		Tax Payments				Transfer Receipts			
	Net Tax Payment	Labor Income Taxes	Capital Income Taxes	Payroll Taxes	Excise Taxes	OASDI	Medicare	Medicaid	Welfare
0	77.40	33.5	9.0	34.3	31.5	7.2	4.7	14.9	4.2
5	95.70	41.6	11.2	42.8	36.6	8.8	5.7	16.7	5.2
10	119.50	52.1	14.3	53.9	42.5	10.6	7.2	19.1	6.5
15	149.10	65.1	18.1	67.8	48.6	12.1	8.8	21.5	8.1
20	182.20	79.5	23.5	83.6	53.4	13.7	10.9	23.5	9.7
25	196.20	86.0	27.9	90.6	53.5	16.4	12.7	22.7	10.1
30	196.80	86.3	33.7	90.2	52.7	19.9	15.0	21.5	9.8
35	189.00	82.9	40.7	86.0	51.4	24.6	17.8	20.4	9.2
40	171.20	76.0	46.6	78.6	50.4	30.8	21.6	19.3	8.7
45	139.20	65.1	50.2	67.4	47.7	38.8	26.1	18.2	8.1
50	93.70	50.8	51.3	52.9	43.7	49.3	31.6	16.5	7.6
55	37.50	34.6	49.7	36.3	38.7	62.8	37.4	14.6	7.0
60	−25.50	18.6	46.3	19.5	32.9	80.1	43.9	12.6	6.3
65	−77.70	7.4	41.2	7.5	27.5	91.8	53.3	10.6	5.7
70	−89.20	3.2	33.0	3.3	22.2	85.0	51.6	9.3	5.1
75	−87.90	1.6	22.4	1.7	16.9	71.7	46.1	8.5	4.2
80	−77.20	0.9	11.2	1.0	11.9	54.8	37.4	6.9	3.1
85	−68.30	0.7	0.0	0.7	8.0	42.6	26.8	6.1	2.1
90	−53.80	0.5	0.0	0.5	6.3	33.7	21.1	4.7	1.7

NOTE: The absolute net tax of future males is 134.6.

The imbalance in generational policy is 71.9 percent.

SOURCE: Authors' calculations.

Table 7.2 U.S. Female Generational Accounts (present values in thousands of 1995 dollars, $r = .06, g = .012$)

	Tax Payments					Transfer Receipts			
Age in 1995	Net Tax Payment	Capital Income Taxes	Income Taxes	Payroll Taxes	Excise Taxes	OASDI	Medicare	Medicaid	Welfare
0	51.9	19.4	9.5	20.9	30.4	6.8	5.0	9.8	6.8
5	63.4	24.1	11.9	26.1	35.2	8.3	6.1	10.8	8.5
10	78.1	30.2	15.1	32.9	40.5	10.0	7.7	12.3	10.6
15	95.7	37.7	19.3	41.3	45.6	11.3	9.5	13.9	13.5
20	115.0	45.7	24.8	50.7	49.8	12.7	11.7	14.9	16.8
25	122.6	48.1	30.3	53.7	50.4	15.3	13.7	15.2	15.7
30	120.7	46.2	36.2	51.6	50.1	18.6	16.1	15.6	13.2
35	113.8	42.8	42.3	47.9	49.8	23.0	19.1	16.1	10.8
40	99.0	38.2	46.3	43.0	48.6	28.8	22.9	16.7	8.7
45	72.8	31.6	47.7	35.7	46.2	36.5	27.5	17.5	7.0
50	37.4	23.6	46.8	26.9	42.3	46.9	33.1	16.5	5.6
55	−5.2	15.0	44.8	17.2	37.6	60.6	39.2	15.3	4.8
60	−52.0	7.6	41.6	8.7	32.4	78.6	45.4	14.1	4.2
65	−91.2	2.7	35.6	3.1	27.1	89.3	53.7	12.8	3.8
70	−101.0	1.0	25.3	1.2	22.2	83.4	51.8	12.1	3.4
75	−101.0	0.5	14.1	0.6	16.9	71.6	46.7	11.8	2.9
80	−90.2	0.3	5.3	0.3	12.4	57.2	38.7	10.1	2.4
85	−73.5	0.1	0.0	0.1	9.4	43.5	28.4	9.4	1.9
90	−55.8	0.1	0.0	0.1	7.2	33.2	21.5	7.0	1.5

NOTE: The absolute net tax of future females is 90.2.

SOURCE: Authors' calculations.

projections used in the accounts are those prevailing as of late fall 1998. The tables show the remaining lifetime net tax payments of every fifth male and female cohort alive in 1995. The figures are based on a 6 percent real discount rate and a 1.2 percent rate of labor productivity growth.[4] All government (local, state, and federal) taxes and transfer payments are included in the analysis.

Consider 40-year-old males. Their remaining lifetime net tax payment is $171,200. This is much higher than the $77,400 in net taxes owed, in present value, by newborn males, because these newborn males are many years away from paying much in the way of taxes. On the other hand, it's smaller than the $196,800 account of 30-year-old males, who have almost all of their peak tax-paying years ahead of them and who are farther away, in time, from receiving significant transfers in the form of Social Security, Medicare, and Medicaid benefits. Compared to 40-year-old males—and, indeed, any males under age 55—males 60 and older are, on average, net recipients of the government's largess. Seventy-year-old males, for example, can expect to receive an average of $89,200 from the government in benefits above and beyond what they can expect to pay in future taxes.

The female generational accounts share the same general age pattern as do the male accounts, but the size of the accounts is smaller for females than for males. Female newborns face a $51,900 lifetime net tax bill compared with $77,400 for male newborns. And female 70-year-olds can look forward to receiving $101,000 over the remainder of their lives from the fiscal system, compared to $89,200 for 70-year-old males. The lower accounts for newborn females than for newborn males reflect females' projected lower labor earnings and lower tax payments over their work span. The larger net transfers owed to 70-year-old females compared to 70-year-old males reflect the longer expected life span of females.

The accounts for future males also exceed those for future females in accordance with our assumption used in the calculations that the ratio of female to male accounts for future generations equals the ratio prevailing for newborns. Future males can anticipate receiving a $134,600 growth-adjusted lifetime net tax bill upon their arrival on earth. For future females the bill is $90,200. Again, the growth adjustment refers to the assumption that each generation born in the future makes a 1.2 percent higher absolute lifetime net tax payment than does the generation coming before it, where 1.2 percent is the assumed rate of labor productivity growth.

Since the accounts for newborn males and females are $77,400 and $51,900, respectively, the growth-adjusted accounts for future generations are 72 percent larger than those of newborns. The size of the generational imbalance can also be described in terms of lifetime net tax rates. As discussed in Gokhale, Page, and Sturrock (1999), male and female newborns face a collective projected lifetime net tax bill equal to 28.6 percent of their projected lifetime labor earnings. For future generations, the corresponding projected lifetime net tax rate is 49.2 percent—or 1.72 times the tax rate facing newborns! Since most current older and working generations will also face lifetime net tax rates of roughly 30 percent, the status quo policy entertained in tables 7.1 and 7.2 entails a policy of much higher rates of lifetime net taxation of future than of current generations.

This represents an enormous imbalance in U.S. generational policy. Forcing future generations to pay lifetime net tax rates that are 72 percent higher than those facing current generations is not only highly inequitable; it's also likely to be economically infeasible. Recall that the 49.2 percent lifetime net tax rate is a net tax and that it also represents an average, rather than a marginal, tax rate. The marginal gross tax rates on various economic activities that the government might try to impose in order to collect a 49.2 percent average net tax rate could well be so high as to preclude actually collecting this net tax; that is, sky-high marginal tax rates could so dissuade future generations from working and saving, that the government finds itself unable to collect the net tax revenue it needs to satisfy its intertemporal budget constraint.

Medicare and U.S. Generational Accounts

Tables 7.1 and 7.2 break down the generational accounts of current generations into their various tax and transfer components. The tax components are labor income taxes, capital income taxes, payroll taxes, and excise taxes. The transfer components are OASDI (Social Security), Medicare, Medicaid, and welfare. The welfare category includes all non-OASDI, Medicare, and Medicaid transfers.

Medicare is clearly a very important transfer component. Indeed, for most generations, it represents the second largest transfer component after Social Security benefits. Take 70-year-olds. The present value of the projected Medicare transfer to males in this age group is $51,600. For equally aged females, it's $51,800. This is about five-eighths of the corresponding Social Security transfer. It's also over four

Table 7.3 1995 Scaled Generational Accounts for Six OECD Countries in Thousands of 1995 U.S. Dollars

Generations	**United States**	**Japan**	**Germany**	**Italy**	**Canada**	**France**
0	86.3	175.1	221.8	155.2	145.3	194.5
5	102.0	206.7	261.2	180.6	166.2	246.1
10	121.7	244.3	314.2	209.4	194.1	294.5
15	144.6	288.0	382.0	242.4	225.9	339.9
20	168.7	339.6	448.4	262.9	254.2	390.8
25	175.4	360.4	416.3	250.5	234.6	418.2
30	170.0	363.6	365.3	210.9	241.5	377.0
35	157.5	350.9	301.6	154.2	211.0	311.6
40	135.7	322.1	215.2	86.4	175.4	214.1
45	101.3	278.0	126.3	14.5	126.3	99.5
50	56.4	211.4	−5.6	−63.6	66.2	−16.0
55	4.0	120.9	−132.9	−140.1	7.4	−172.9
60	51.7	14.5	−246.8	−192.9	−57.9	−252.9
65	96.0	−58.2	−277.8	−187.9	−108.2	−256.6
70	104.6	−54.7	−242.9	−159.6	−113.8	−194.5
75	101.9	−11.0	−201.9	−128.7	−109.3	−208.1
80	89.5	−32.6	−147.3	−98.1	−103.3	−120.5
85	74.4	−22.2	−91.4	−71.6	−88.6	−132.1
90	−56.7	−11.8	−4.3	−10.1	−14.0	−121.2
Future Generations	130.4	471.6	425.8	359.8	145.6	286.0
Generational Imbalance						
Absolute	44.1	296.5	204.0	204.6	0.3	91.5
In percent	51.1	169.3	92.0	131.8	0.0	47.1

SOURCE: Kotlikoff and Leibfritz (1999).

times larger than the corresponding Medicaid transfer. Since the generational accounts of 70-year-old males and females are −\$89,200 and −\$101,000, respectively, Medicare is responsible for more than half of the remaining lifetime net transfer being made to this cohort.

Even though Medicare benefits are only available to disabled workers prior to age 65, the program's net transfers loom quite large for young and middle-aged workers. Take 45-year-olds. Their projected Medicare transfer exceeds \$25,000 in present value. These transfers, in conjunction with the Social Security transfer, exceed the present value of the generation's projected future payroll taxes; that is, this generation has a larger stake in maintaining the pay-as-you-go financed Social Security and Medicare programs than it does in eliminating them.

IV. Comparing U.S. Generational Accounts to Those of Other Developed Countries

Table 7.3, gleaned from Kotlikoff and Leibfritz (1999), compares U.S. generational accounts with those of Japan, Germany, Italy, Canada, and France. All table 7.3 entries are in 1995 dollars. Unlike tables 7.1 and 7.2, which incorporate a 6 percent discount rate and a 1.2 percent labor productivity growth rate, table 7.3 assumes a 5 percent discount rate and a 1.5 percent labor productivity growth rate.[5] It also combines males and females in reporting the overall remaining lifetime net tax payment of different generations.

In addition, to ease cross-country comparisons, the generational accounts of all the foreign countries are scaled by the ratio of 1995 U.S. per capita GDP to the country's 1995 per capita GDP. For example, U.S. per capita GDP in 1995 was 1.28 times larger than France's per capita GDP. Hence, the French generational account values were multiplied by 1.28 before being recorded in table 7.3. By scaling the foreign country accounts in this manner, we can immediately consider whether particular cohorts in particular countries have high or low generational accounts compared with those in the United States, after controlling for the relative living standards and levels of economic activity in those countries.

The first thing to notice in table 7.3 is the bottom line, which indicates the percentage imbalance in each country's generational policy. For the United States, there is a 51.1 percent imbalance. Again, this figure differs from the imbalance reported in table 7.1 because of the assumed lower discount rate and the assumed higher labor productivity growth rate. Although the U.S. generational imbalance is sizable, it is actually relatively small compared to the imbalances in Japan, Italy, and Germany. Their imbalances are 169.3 percent, 131.8 percent, and 92.0 percent, respectively. In other words, future Japanese, Italians, and Germans face lifetime net tax rates that, respectively, are 2.7, 2.3, and 1.9 times as large as those now facing newborn Japanese, Italians, and Germans under current policy. In contrast, France's 47.1 percent imbalance is smaller than that of the United States, and Canada's imbalance is essentially zero. Given the discussion above about the lack of a theoretical basis for deficit accounting, it's interesting to note the absence of any positive correlation between the size of these imbalances and the countries' official net debt to GDP ratios. These ratios are .48 for the United States, .10 for Japan, .45 for Germany, 1.10 for Italy, .69 for Canada, and .36 for France. Thus Japan, which has the largest generational imbalance of the six countries, has the smallest debt-to-GDP ratio, and Canada, which has the smallest generational imbalance, has the second largest debt-to-GDP ratio.

The sources of generational imbalance in the various countries differ across the countries. In Japan, the scaled generational accounts of both the young and the old substantially exceed those of young and old Americans. For example, 40-year-olds face remaining lifetime net taxes of $101,300 in the United States, but $322,100 in Japan! And 70-year-old Americans can expect to receive $104,600 in net transfers over the rest of their lives compared with only $54,700 for comparably aged Japanese. These findings would, other things equal, suggest a smaller generational imbalance in Japan than in the United States. But other things aren't equal. The Japanese generational imbalance is greater than that of the United States, in part, because of its level of projected government purchases and, in part, because of its demographics. Japan's population is aging more rapidly and more significantly than that of the United States. In the United States today, there are close to 19 elderly for every 100 workers. In 2030 there will be 37 elderly for every 100 workers. In Japan today there are only about 17 elderly per 100 workers, but in 2030 there will be 45 elderly per 100 workers.

Germany's population will age less rapidly than Japan's but end up with a higher elderly dependency ratio than Japan. In 2030 there will be 49 older Germans for each 100 German workers, compared to about 22 per 100 right now. The timing of Germany's aging coupled with the extremely high level of net taxes it is collecting from current German workers explain why Germany's generational imbalance is less severe than that of either Japan or Italy.

Canada is another interesting case. Projected Canadian demographic change is fairly similar to that of the United States. This point notwithstanding, Canada's intergenerational imbalance is zero, whereas the U.S. imbalance is over 50 percent. The main difference in policy is that Canada is collecting substantially larger net taxes from current Canadian workers than is the United States. For 30-year-olds, for example, the scaled Canadian generational account is $241,500 compared with $170,000 for the United States.

V. Cutting Medicare Benefits to Achieve Generational Balance

Although the imbalance in U.S. generational policy is quite large, it is substantially smaller than it was a couple of years ago. The improvement in the U.S. generational imbalance can be traced to changes in policy that have led to revised fiscal projections and changes in the fiscal projections of the same policies.

Medicare is a prime example. Since 1995 Medicare has been subject to significant legislative changes. A number of the assumptions underlying its projected expenditures have also been reassessed by HCFA. Figure 7.1 presents past and projected future Medicare outlays as a percent of GDP. For years after 1995, the figure shows the Medicare-GDP ratio as projected in 1995 (labeled Pr 1995) and the ratio projected in 1997 (labeled Pr 1997). There is a tremendous difference in

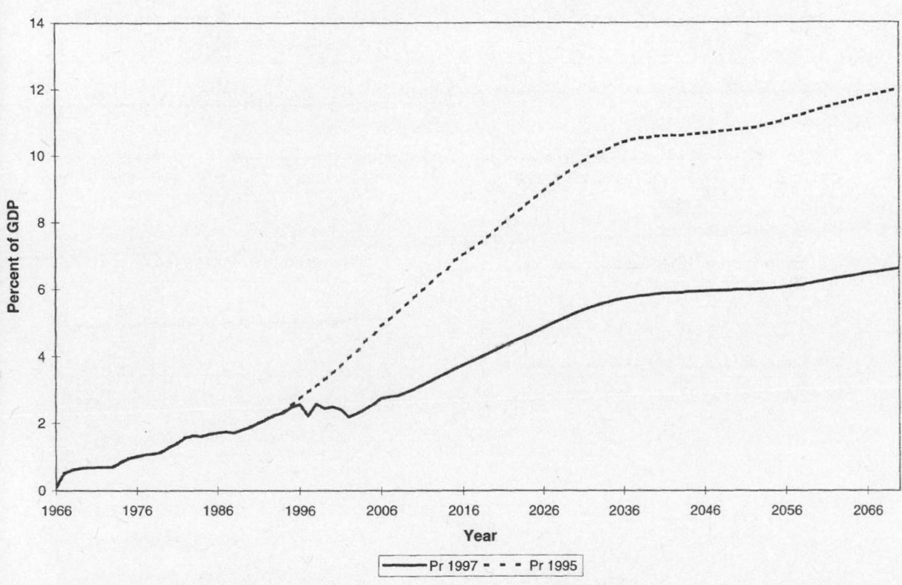

Figure 7.1 Medicare Outlays (1966–1995) and Projections (1996–2070) as a Percentage of GDP

SOURCE: Authors' calculations.

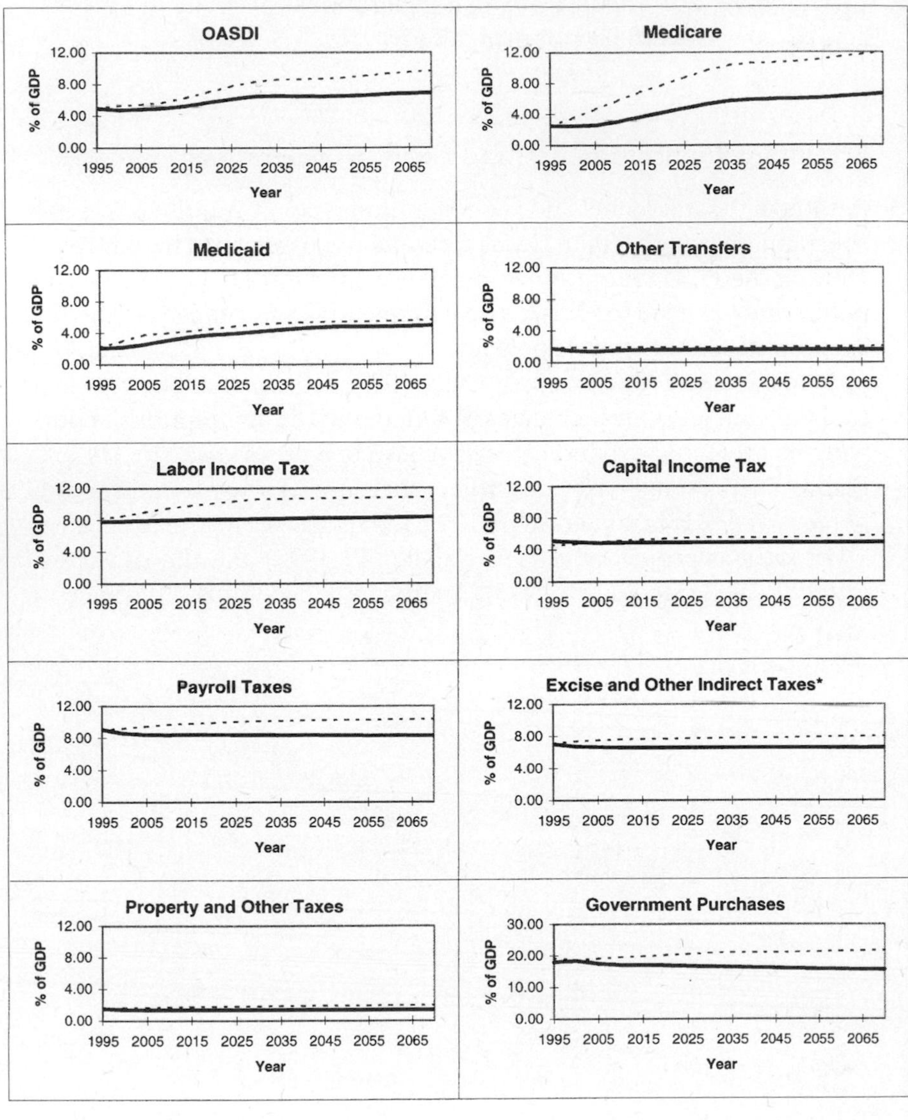

Figure 7.2 Comparison of Projected Budget Aggregates—GA1993 and GA1995

*Excludes property taxes.

Source: OMB, CBO, and authors' calculations.

these two projections, culminating in a variance of more than 5 percentage points in the long-run ratio of Medicare to GDP. Note that current Medicare expenditures are now roughly 2.5 percent of U.S. GDP, so the revision in the government's long-run forecast of the size of this program amounts to the equivalent of two expenditure programs that are each as large, relative to the U.S. economy, as the current Medicare program!

Figure 7.2 repeats figure 7.1 but also shows the revisions between 1995 and 1997 in projections of different taxes, transfer programs, and government purchases relative to GDP. Although the revisions in Medicare projections are the most dramatic, the 1997 projections also incorporate much lower projected future OASDI expenditures and government purchases. They also incorporate significantly lower projected future government labor income and payroll tax receipts. In the case of labor income taxes, there is a difference of over 3 percentage points in the long-run projected ratio of these receipts to GDP.

The lower long-run Medicare projections appear, in large part, to be inspired by success in the past couple of years in maintaining the level of Medicare expenditures relative to GDP. Part of this success stems from shifting a portion of the Medicare population into health maintenance organizations and other managed care programs. Whether or not the improvements in the projections of long-run Medicare expenditures are justified, it's clear that there is a great deal of uncertainty about future Medicare expenditures and that future generations can ill afford any long-term forecasting mistakes on the part of current policy makers. Given how much the government has changed its long-term Medicare forecast in just the past two years, one could argue that the government should err on the conservative side in using Medicare forecasts to help assess the imbalance in U.S. generational policy.

Achieving Generational Balance via Medicare Cuts

Table 7.4 examines the permanent cuts in Medicare benefits that could be used to achieve generational balance, by which we mean equalizing the lifetime net tax rates of current newborns and future generations. The table considers baseline (current) policy as well as three other policies: (1) limiting government purchases after the turn of the century to the same real amount as that spent in 2000; (2) reducing the annual real growth rate of Medicare and Medicaid expenditures per beneficiary by

Table 7.4 Eliminating the U.S. Generational Policy Imbalance via Medicare Cuts Policy

	Baseline	Limit Gov. Expenditures	Limit Medical Expenditures	Limit Gov. Purchases and Medical Expenditures
Policy Begins in 1998				
Percentage cut	68.0	52.8	31.0	11.1
Initial dollar cut	239.0	185.7	108.9	39.1
Equalized Net Tax Rate	30.1	29.8	31.4	31.1
Policy Begins in 2003				
Percentage cut	77.6	60.3	36.8	13.2
Initial dollar cut	299.1	232.4	141.9	51.0
Equalized Net Tax Rate	30.3	29.9	31.5	31.1
Policy Begins in 2016				
Percentage cut	111.3	86.5	55.5	19.9
Initial dollar cut	828.5	643.7	413.1	148.4
Equalized Net Tax Rate	31.0	30.5	31.8	31.2

SOURCE: Authors' calculations.

2 percentage points between now and 2003 and permitting real expenditures per beneficiary on these programs to grow after 2003 at the growth rate of labor productivity; and (3) simultaneously engaging in policies (1) and (2). The table also considers initiating the cuts in Medicare at three different dates: 1998, 2003, and 2016.

Table 7.4 shows the requisite permanent percentage cut in Medicare benefits needed to achieve generational balance given the policy in place and the start date for the cut. It also shows the absolute Medicare spending cut in billions of 1995 dollars in the first year the policy is initiated. Finally, the table shows the common lifetime net tax rate that will face future and newborn generations once the specified policy is enacted.

Under baseline policy, the United States can achieve generational balance by either (1) permanently cutting Medicare by 68 percent starting right now; (2) waiting five years and permanently cutting Medicare by 78 percent; or (3) waiting until 2016 and finding out that even the total elimination of the program is insufficient to produce generational balance. The simple arithmetic of generational accounting makes time a grim reaper. The longer the government waits to administer its painful medicine, the more cohorts who escape having to take that medicine and the more medicine that needs to be taken by those cohorts who are left behind.

In terms of its impact on the conventional budget deficit, achieving generational balance via an immediate and permanent cut in Medicare would entail running close to a $250 billion surplus this year and for many years into the future. This is a vast sum compared to the current official $8 billion surplus that our politicians are (1) holding up as a sign of prudent fiscal management and (2) contemplating spending.

Restraining government purchases is one of many ways of limiting requisite Medicare cuts. But even if real federal purchases were held absolutely fixed after 2000, an immediate and permanent 53 percent cut in Medicare spending would still be needed to achieve generational balance. This is a remarkable finding. Holding federal purchases fixed in real terms as the economy continues to grow means that the federal government is asymptotically eliminated. But even the eventual effective elimination of general federal government appears to be far too little too late to rescue the next generation. Another way to try to avoid immediate Medicare cuts is simply to slow the growth of its expenditures as well as those of Medicaid. The third column of table 7.4 contemplates such a policy. Unfortunately, slowing down health care spending through 2003 and allowing Medicare and Medicaid benefits per beneficiary to grow no faster than the rate of labor productivity growth also fall far short of what is needed for generational equity. Even with such a slow-growth policy, the initial level of Medicare would need to be reduced by almost one-third. Indeed, an immediate and permanent 11 percent cut in Medicare benefits is needed even if (1) the federal government is allowed to slowly dematerialize and (2) the growth of health care spending is finally brought under control.

VI. Conclusion

Recent U.S. policy changes and more optimistic fiscal forecasts have significantly improved the long-term fiscal prospects of the country. Nevertheless, these prospects remain dismal. Unless U.S. fiscal policy changes by a lot and very soon, our descendants will face rates of lifetime net taxation that are 70 percent higher than those we now face. They will, on average, find themselves paying one of every two dollars they earn to a local, state, or federal government in net taxes.

Encumbering our progeny with a fiscal burden of this magnitude, apart from the question of its morality, could well prove economically infeasible. As a host of countries in Latin America and Eastern Europe know all too well, there is a limit to the amount of resources governments can extract from their economies. Once that limit is reached, governments find themselves forced to print money to try to pay their bills. Hyperinflation, the gradual disappearance of the formal sector, anemic national saving, meager rates of domestic investment, and economic stagnation are the legacies of trying to take from the private sector more than it's able or willing to give.

A number of factors, besides current and projected Medicare spending, are responsible for the imbalance in U.S. generational policy. But the ongoing excessive growth of Medicare benefits is certainly a key culprit. Achieving generational balance solely by cutting Medicare benefits is feasible but would require cutting over two-thirds of the program's expenditures assuming the cuts were made today. If one waits five years before cutting Medicare, four-fifths of the program would have to be slashed. Clearly, Medicare cuts of this magnitude are unlikely to happen; but however we resolve our severe crisis in U.S. generational policy, it's clear that significant reductions in Medicare spending will be a major part of the story.

Notes

1. Some of our recent generational accounting (for example, Kotlikoff and Leibfritz 1999) also treats educational expenditures as a transfer payment.

2. Here are just six examples of the different ways one can describe a dollar given this year to the government: (1) a $1 tax; (2) a $1 loan to the government; (3) a $2 loan to the government less the receipt of a $1 transfer payment; (4) a $5,000,000 loan to the government less the receipt of a $4,999,999 transfer payment; (5) a $2 tax less a $1 loan received from the government; (6) a $999 tax less a $998 loan received from the government. Compared to case (1), using the language in the other cases will generate the following increases in this year's official debt: (2) $1, (3) $2, (4) $5,000,000, (5) −$1, and (6) −$998.

3. For example, in estimating average values of future payroll tax payments by age and sex, we use a cross-section-relative payroll-tax profile that we obtain from the latest available Current Population Survey. Assuming, as we do, that this profile will hold for future years may be introducing a bias in the calculation of generational accounts in so far as the shape of this profile has a predictable trend. Further research is needed to address this issue.

4. In applying this labor productivity growth rate to the average values of real taxes and transfers, we are implicitly assuming that the annual real labor compensation, upon which average real taxes and transfers are based, rises at this same growth rate. One could refine these calculations by entertaining separate growth rates in real wages per hour and in total hours worked per year.

5. This somewhat higher labor productivity growth rate was used because it seemed to better accord with historical labor productivity growth averaged across all the countries included in the studied.

References

Auerbach, Alan J., Jagadeesh Gokhale, and Laurence J. Kotlikoff. 1991. "Generational Accounts: A Meaningful Alternative to Deficit Accounting." In *Tax Policy and the Economy 5,* edited by D. Bradford. Cambridge: MIT Press, pp. 55–110.

———. 1995. "Restoring Generational Balance in U.S. Fiscal Policy: What Will It Take?" Federal Reserve Bank of Cleveland, *Economic Review* 31 (1): 2–12.

Auerbach, Alan J., and Laurence J. Kotlikoff. 1999. "The Methodology of Generational Accounting." In *Generational Accounting around the World,* edited by Alan J. Auerbach, Laurence J. Kotlikoff, and Willi Leibfritz. Chicago: Chicago University Press.

Congressional Budget Office. 1995. *Who Pays and When: An Assessment of Generational Accounting.* Washington, D.C.: U.S. Government Printing Office.

Gokhale, Jagadeesh, Benjamin R. Page, and John R. Sturrock. 1999. "Generational Accounts for the U.S.: An Update." In *Generational Accounting around the World,* edited by Alan J. Auerbach, Laurence J. Kotlikoff, and Willi Leibfritz. Chicago: Chicago University Press.

Kotlikoff, Laurence J. 1992. *Generational Accounting.* New York: The Free Press.

Kotlikoff, Laurence J., and Willi Leibfritz. 1999. "An International Comparison of Generational Accounts." In *Generational Accounting around the World,* edited by Alan J. Auerbach, Laurence J. Kotlikoff, and Willi Leibfritz. Chicago: Chicago University Press.

Chapter Eight

Comment: Asking the Right Questions in the Medicare Reform Debate

Kevin M. Murphy

In discussing the contributions by Frank A. Sloan and Donald H. Taylor Jr., David M. Cutler, and Jagadeesh Gokhale and Laurence J. Kotlikoff, it is important to consider the general kind of ideas and issues that are embodied in their papers. First of all, Cutler has the right idea with his statement "We have to ask the right questions," although I do not think he did ask the right questions, as I discuss below. At the outset, one has to make a distinction between two terms: Medicare and medical care. These are clearly not synonyms, but much of the discussion concerning Medicare seems to treat them as if they are.

An example of how misinterpreting the distinction between Medicare and medical care can lead to fuzzy thinking is embodied in the question posed in Cutler's chapter: "Would you prefer today's Medicare system to the Medicare system of 1970?" If answered no, it cannot be proven wrong by showing that today's medical care is better than the medical care from 1970. The question is about Medicare and the answer concerns medical care. Had the original question been about medical care, a different answer would have been given. That is to say, consider somebody who proposes that Medicare be abolished. Does this mean that person wants to abolish *medical care*? If one wanted to go back to 1900 medical care, does this mean they want to go back and get bled every six months to make them feel better? Of course not.

Kevin M. Murphy is the George Pratt Shultz Professor of Business Economics and Industrial Relations at the University of Chicago.

Cutler makes the point that since the inception of Medicare, both the life expectancy and the general health status of the elderly have improved. The notion that Medicare is responsible for the improvement we have seen over the last several decades, even if the facts were all there, is rather dubious. There is simply much more going on than just the institutional change that has resulted in increased use of the health care system by the elderly.

What Are the Facts?

Asking the right questions about Medicare as a public policy issue is a top priority; and this brings about a second question, which is a continuing theme in all of the chapters: What are the facts? What has happened over time? Several of the authors show that medical expenditures have grown not necessarily as a result of inflation, per se, but as a result of increased quantity of health care consumed.

Cutler, for example, contrasts the growth in health care expenditures to the growth in expenditures on computers. Like health care, computer consumption has grown. Total expenditures on computers have grown even in a period of falling prices. In determining whether the increase in per capita Medicare spending has been worth it, Cutler suggests that we have to look at the benefits. But it is more than that. Returning to the computer example, growing expenditures is not considered to be a problem because the people getting the benefits are paying the costs. Choosing to spend ten times more on computers today than what you spent before is not a problem as long as you pay from your own pocket.

This relates to the point made in Gokhale and Kotlikoff's chapter. The big policy issue is who is paying for the elderly's medical care. To a large extent this is the correct conclusion. But it is not necessarily just because of the intergenerational imbalance. The fundamental issue is who is paying for medical care, and a key question is whether the financing arrangements lead to excess consumption. So it is critical to step back for a moment and think about the issues and the facts. The facts are that medical care expenditures were growing rapidly and the growth was coming from growth in quantity. Second, over the same time period, the payments for that consumption were coming from the public. While it is clear that there has been considerable expenditure growth in the Medicare system, there has also been a lot of growth in other parts of the health care system as well; Cutler and Victor R. Fuchs both point to the growth in the private sector. Nonetheless, when considering Medicare, one of the big issues is who is footing the bill.

Intergenerational Considerations

In thinking about footing the bill for Medicare and the fact that Medicare has been growing, we should consider the work of Paul Samuelson on Social Security. His analysis concludes that the growth in the system compared to the rate of interest determines who pays. This is the right way to think about the Medicare issue: it doesn't determine whether it's efficient or inefficient; it just determines who's paying. If expenditures are growing at the interest rate, then the system does not charge one group at the expense of the other. If the population is also growing, then each generation gets benefits back that are greater than what they paid into the system in tax payments.

Does the fact that individuals receive an amount equal to their tax payments plus interest mean there is no cost? No, the cost is the same, regardless of the method of finance. It just means more of the cost is being passed on to future generations. Gokhale and Kotlikoff are right in suggesting that the debts being imposed on future generations need to be considered today. They talk about it as a generational imbalance measured by a comparison of the costs being imposed on today's young as opposed to the costs that are being imposed on future young.

In Gokhale and Kotlikoff's work, Canada looks better than the United States, for example, in the costs imposed on future generations. But looking at the absolute cost being imposed on future young, instead, the two countries are almost the same. This comparison is not quite fair because there are other government services built into those numbers that somehow would have to be standardized out. To be able to see the costs net of "pay for services at time rendered" would be a useful modification to this methodology. Regardless, what is far more important than just the imbalance in numbers is the magnitude of some of the debts. In some countries children are born owing $450,000. Is such a debt fair? If the service component of government is standardized out, fair would be zero. Fairness implies that you pay for what you use. So, the amount of net taxes implied by such systems is rather enormous.

The chapters contained in this volume are about theories, about things like adverse selection, moral hazard, and market failure. These issues have nothing to do with the intergenerational question. That is, one cannot justify the intergenerational imbalance on the basis of a theory about adverse selection or moral hazard or whatever. So it seems one of the clearest roads to go down—and the road that Gokhale and Kotlikoff are suggesting—is one of trying to handle the intergenerational imbalance. The imbalance can be rectified by raising taxes and raising taxes right away. But that only goes part way. Cutting benefits, of course, does a better job because it spreads the burden over a wider range of individuals.

The amount of generational imbalance that we have in the current system is really not so much a function of policy choices up until now, but is rather an inherent characteristic of the pay-as-you-go system. Any pay-as-you-go system is going to have an enormous burden placed on future generations. There is this misconception: Everybody always remembers Samuelson. The Samuelson result says that when the growth of the economy is close to the interest rate, it is beneficial to run a pay-as-you-go system. This is only true if the growth goes on forever. In fact, growth could continue indefinitely, but as soon as it stops, nothing has been gained for the entire time period. It is not optimal to run that kind of system until the point is reached where the growth rate falls down to the rate of interest and then switch—because at that time it all comes due.

The only Ponzi scheme that ever works is the one that is never called. If you ever get called on your pyramid, you pay the full price. And that is the issue right now. The longer we run the pyramid scheme, the bigger the full price that is going to come due and the smaller the number of people that are going to bear the consequences. It is incomprehensible that we continue with the current generational transfer scheme.

Moral Hazard and Adverse Selection

Returning to the issue of expenditure growth, a more fundamental issue is at work here. Again, is the growth in expenditures so important? Typically, economists are neutral on how individuals allocate their budgets, but in the case of Medicare, there are a couple of issues: Are beneficiaries spending other people's money? One way to think about this is in the generational sense. Are today's elderly spending the future generation's money? That is clearly a problem. Suppose this is fixed; is that the end of the story? The answer is no, in that as long as the system is public, anytime a beneficiary draws from the system, the payments come out of somebody else's pocket.

Spending somebody else's money is also true of third-party payment schemes. But there is a difference between third-party private schemes and the government schemes. First, third-party schemes do not allow the older generation to impose the cost on the young. In a third-party scheme, the members of the group bear the cost. Secondly, in a private scheme, if there is a moral hazard problem where beneficiaries do not bear the cost of excess consumption, do they at least get to choose how much of a moral hazard problem they are willing to endure? Greater insurance arises with moral hazard at the expense of excess consumption. But with private contracting, the trade-off between the consequences of moral hazard and the benefits of insurance tends to produce positive results.

Can the same be said when adverse selection is considered? Adverse selection brings up the issue of a single mandatory policy for everybody. But even in this context, two elements that define differences across people must be considered. There are the elements that are known by the market and the elements that are unknown by the market. Trying to handle the ones that are unknown by the market in order to manage adverse selection by having one policy for everybody actually aggravates the other problem. With one policy and one price for everybody, what happens? Given that sellers cannot charge higher prices to higher-risk beneficiaries, they resort to risk-based screening—whereas with a free market system, screening would not be a problem. Insurers would serve higher-risk applicants, but the price would be high. The basic point is that adverse selection problems are different and occur for different reasons, depending on whether the information is known to the individual or known to the market.

Why not just let the market act on all the available information? What would the cost be? The cost of allowing the market to act on its information is that some insurance possibilities are forgone. The market can no longer insure against known conditions because the cost of known conditions is taken into account in individual-specific prices. How is this avoided? One way is to contract early enough, so that conditions are not known to either party when the contract begins. Ideally, the contract begins at birth, but such a contract has its own problems.

Consider writing a contract fifty years ago that could have adapted to new medical technologies like today's angioplasty. Writing such a contract that far in advance is pretty difficult, so early contracting is not necessarily the catch-all solution.

But other ways exist. One is to try to distinguish two types of expenditures that people incur. Greater expenditures can result from the desire to purchase a more elaborate plan or can be the result of greater risks. The policy issue is then one of separating between the two, by subsidizing beneficiaries' payments as a function of risk but not subsidizing payments as a function of whether beneficiaries want a Cadillac or a Yugo health plan. This is an important element to get at in any system. Instinctively, one would be to try to get people signed up early but not necessarily really early. Those contracts are too hard to write. Ideally, the contract would be signed sometime before retirement.

Conclusion

There is also another issue at work here. Even after addressing the intergenerational issue and after tackling the moral hazard and adverse selection questions, there is the old problem of getting people to save for the future. People think of socialization of health care as a solution to that question. But is socialization of health care really the *cause* of that problem? Let's say everybody is sent off on a spacecraft, given a food supply, and each provided with a little capsule. Would a time-release food supply that would keep them from eating it up before they got to their destination be necessary? No. But now suppose that they are all on the same spacecraft and the refrigerator is downstairs. What would happen? A time-release lock on the refrigerator, which opens the door only once in a while, may be a good idea. Just a little food for thought in terms of where we are headed.

So in concluding a discussion of these broad issues of Medicare reform, it is crucial to ask the right questions. But it is also crucial to distinguish between medical care and Medicare. The two are not synonymous. When we think about solutions, we think about solutions that involve the most difficult question: What is the right level of service? Should we have a Cadillac plan, which is very expensive and takes advantage of all the latest technology? Or should we have the Yugo plan? Why is that question being asked? That question is not asked for

Cadillacs and Yugos. Adverse selection and moral hazard are also relevant issues but are not central. When increasing the labor supply of the elderly or when other things are being considered as public policy choices, then I think the problem is reversed. Much of the labor supply behavior of the elderly has more to do with public policy problems than with public policy solutions.

Chapter Nine

Paying for Medicare in the Twenty-first Century

Andrew J. Rettenmaier and Thomas R. Saving

As we near the beginning of the twenty-first century, Medicare is headed toward a precipice. Under the current program and financing, the unfunded liability of Medicare—even under conservative assumptions—exceeds $8 trillion. This unfunded liability is more than two times the current national debt and at least 50 percent greater than the more discussed Social Security unfunded liability. What is interesting is that the financial precipice was foreseen by the members of Congress who passed the legislation in 1965. At that time, key members of Congress saw medical expenditures growing at rates that exceeded the growth in earnings. Because the program was to be financed with payroll taxes, congressional leaders predicted that the tax base and tax rate would have to be raised to keep pace with the program's growth. This is exactly what happened over the program's first three decades. In the future, further tax increases or benefit cuts will be necessary. Given the magnitude of the unfunded liability, an immediate tax increase of 72 percent is necessary to make the system solvent; therefore, the system requires more than minor changes at this point. While it is easy to look back and wonder why the program ever won approval in light of the expected financing problems, the hard task is to frame a fundamental reform that moves the program toward a sustainable solution.

For long-term success, Medicare reform must address three aspects of the Medicare program that have worked together to get us to the cur-

Dr. Andrew J. Rettenmaier is a research associate at the Private Enterprise Research Center, Texas A&M University.

Dr. Thomas R. Saving heads the Private Enterprise Research Center, Texas A&M University. A University Distinguished Professor of Economics at Texas A&M University, he also holds the Jeff Montgomery Professorship in Economics.

rent situation: a payment scheme insuring that users of the system care little about what it costs, a financing system involving generational transfers as its principal source of revenue, and Congress's penchant of subsidizing "worthy" causes with any funds that appear available. The first issue is shared with the larger medical insurance market. A majority of beneficiaries supplement Medicare with Medigap policies, which produce first-dollar coverage and the accompanying problems of high usage and expenditure growth. The financing system is vulnerable because it is sensitive to generational size shocks, like the baby boom generation. Even with a stable population, if per capita benefits grow at rates that exceed earnings growth, transfer payment financing will require raising tax rates. Furthermore, as long as the program's revenues remain under congressional control, there will exist incentives to spend any surplus funds, either explicitly from the Medicare Trust Fund or implicitly through greater expenditures elsewhere in the budget. In this chapter we address each of these problems and suggest a solution that relies on a gradual transition to prefunded retirement health insurance through individual accounts.

Who Pays and the Escalating per Capita Cost of Medicare

By lowering the price of additional medical care expenditures, insurance increases expenditures above the level that would be consumed in its absence. Consider the difference between the full-page grocery store ads that appear in every daily newspaper and ads touting hospitals or health care providers. The grocery store ads, no matter in what city they appear, are dominated by one thing: the price of the advertised goods. The health care industry also advertises, but in contrast to the grocery store ads, price is seldom, if ever, mentioned. Rather, hospital and medical clinic advertisements focus on the quality of care.

Why is price the principal component of advertising for the grocery supermarket and never mentioned in ads for hospital or medical clinics? The reason is simple and is a major factor in the escalating per capita cost of Medicare: the majority of consumers of medical care are not concerned about its cost because they are not paying for it—at least not directly. Because buyers are not concerned with what medical care costs, the sellers of medical care do not have the incentive to keep cost down. Demanders are happy to demand state-of-the-art care, and suppliers are all too happy to supply it.

In 1997 over 95 percent of all payments to hospitals were from sources other than the recipients of hospital services. For physicians services, almost 85 percent of all 1997 payments were not paid by patients. Even for dental services and prescription drugs—relative newcomers to the prepaid insurance market—less than 50 percent of payments in 1997 were made by the patients. If patients are not paying, who is? The payers are taxpayers, indirectly through Medicare and Medicaid, as well as the patients, indirectly through various medical prepayment plans (commonly known as medical insurance, although the insurance companies simply administer group plans and are not at risk as they would be if insurance were really involved).

To see the impact on the health care industry of who pays, consider the following facts: Over the period from 1960 to 1997, real hospital services expenditures per capita, where patients paid on average only 9 percent of the cost, rose by a factor of 3.4. Over the same period, real physician services expenditures, where patients paid 36 percent of the costs, rose by a factor of 3.5. In contrast, real pharmaceutical expenditures, where patients paid 68 percent of the cost, only rose by a factor of 2.5. Similarly, the real cost of dental care per person, where on average 72 percent of payments were made out-of-pocket, rose by a factor of 2.2. These are powerful facts that relate real increases in costs of medical care to whether or not buyers are concerned with what it costs.[1]

The Tragedy of Medicare Financing

When the Social Security Act was passed in 1935, it was envisioned that the system would be prefunded by those working so that when they retired there would be enough in the "Old-Age Reserve Account" to pay for their retirement.[2] Through a combination of failure to enact the programmed tax increases, premature initiation of payments to retirees, and expansion of benefits, the program came to rely on pay-as-you-go financing. The combined Social Security Trust Fund is estimated to be bankrupt by the year 2032. When Medicare was passed and the Medicare Trust Fund was established, there was never any pretense that the funds in the trust fund would be adequate to pay for the health care expenditures of the covered population. Not surprisingly then, the bankruptcy of the Medicare Trust Fund is expected by the year 2008.

As bad as all this sounds, the real issue may be even worse. The

Social Security and Medicare Trust Funds—indeed, all government trust funds—are not trust funds at all. A trust fund, in its common usage, means resources put away to meet some future contingency. The resources in the government trust funds are composed entirely of promises by the government to use future tax revenues to pay for future expenditures: these promises are not the source of the future revenue.

To better see the relation between what a trust fund contains and that fund's ability to finance the expenditures for which it was established, consider two types of assets in a personal trust fund: bonds issued by entities other than yourself and bonds issued by you. In the former case, the trust fund has as its assets the ownership of income that others are legally obligated to pay to the trust. As a result, when the time comes for the resources in the trust fund to be expended, the availability does not depend on your income at the time, but rather the trust fund represents a prepaid fund. On the other hand, if the trust fund has as its assets newly issued promises to pay by yourself, there is no prepayment.[3]

The Social Security and Medicare Trust Funds both have earmarked revenues from payroll taxes placed in them and, thus, have all the appearances of the first form of a trust fund, a trust fund in which real assets are put away to pay for future expenditures. It is the next step that is crucial to what has happened to these two government trust funds. The government takes the income going into the trust funds and replaces it with its own promises to pay in the future. This is not a problem if the government invests the trust fund revenues in real social overhead capital—such as highways and bridges —which enhances the real productive capacity of the nation. If real capital is greater, when the time comes to use the trust funds, the ability of the government to pay the cost has been enhanced because of real investments made. Unfortunately, even a casual look at the federal budget over the past twenty years indicates that the revenues have all been spent on current consumption, through transfer payments, rather than investment in the nation's capital.

In every sense, the Social Security and Medicare Trust Funds are fiction. There are no real resources put aside to meet the future expenditures that these trust funds were designed to insure. But in another sense, this fact does not matter. All that really matters is whether or not the nation is willing to tighten its belt and pay for the real resources it will take to continue to provide for the retirement and health care of elderly citizens as the population of the elderly grows. If it is not willing to do this belt tightening—and there is little evidence that the federal government is ready to mend its spendthrift ways—then individuals will have to tighten their belts. The belt tightening can begin now with restructuring Social Security and Medicare in such a way that individuals invest in real capital as they save for retirement.

The Worthy-Cause Effect

Because of the incentives inherent in federal programs, the programs tend to expand rather than contract. Medicare is a good example of this expansion. In spite of the precarious long-term financial status of Medicare, by 1972 Congress was already finding worthy causes on which to spend the trust fund balance. These causes were in three areas: an expansion of those eligible to receive Medicare benefits, an expansion of the benefits themselves, and other nonservice but health care related expenditures.

Legislation approved in 1972 extended Medicare coverage to disabled persons under age 65 who were eligible for benefits under Social Security or Railroad Retirement and to certain other individuals under age 65 suffering end-stage renal disease. Coverage was also extended to any individual not eligible for Medicare as a result of not being eligible for Social Security or Railroad Retirement who was aged 65 or older and enrolled in the voluntary Supplemental Medical Insurance (SMI). Then it was extended to state and local government employees not covered by Social Security. Finally, coverage has been extended to spouses of workers who were not currently covered but would be eligible to be covered, and Medicare has become the secondary payer for individuals and their spouses when their work-supplied health care insurance is exhausted.[4]

Quite possibly the most controversial use of the Medicare Trust Fund has been subsidies to teaching hospitals to aid in the training of medical doctors. This program represents a significant subsidy to hospitals in the program. These funds subsidize both the training of physicians and the use of the hospitals by indigent patients. Both of these uses might be worthy of support; but if they are worthy, it seems that general revenue funds could be made available.

Why a Prepaid System?

Moving to a prepaid system of financing Medicare allows us to undo the damage that the current generational transfer system imposes on the economy. This damage is in the form of a reduction in the nation's capital stock. It is well documented, both theoretically and empirically, that a system guaranteeing the retirement of a working generation by imposing taxes on a future generation reduces the incentive for the working generation to provide for its own retirement. The only way society can provide the consumption goods required for both the working and retired generations is by having a sufficient capital stock. If the current working generation faces reduced incentives to accumulate capital, they will pass on to the next generation a smaller capital stock. This smaller capital stock will produce fewer goods and services, leaving all generations poorer.

We can explore the impact of intergenerational transfers on the capital stock by considering a simple economy where only two generations, one working and one retired, are around at any one time. To set a base for our analysis, we begin with a totally private system in which the working generation provides for its own retirement by buying capital from the retired generation and producing the nation's output, some of which is used to add to the nation's capital stock and to replace any depreciation in the capital stock. The working generation then uses the capital stock it has purchased and any additions it has made to the capital stock to sell to the next working generation. The proceeds from the sale of this capital provide the retired generation with its consumption needs.

In figure 9.1, we illustrate the equilibrium for the working generation in our base economy. The working generation must make decisions between consumption now and consumption after retirement. We show the trade-off for the working generation between consumption in their working years, the horizontal axis, and consumption during their retirement years, the vertical axis, as the curve labeled *PP*. Since the level of the capital stock totally determines the level of retirement consumption, as retirement consumption increases—moving upward along the *PP* curve—the capital stock increases. We show the working generation's tastes for current consumption versus retirement consumption as the convex curve labeled *UU,* denoting the working generation's willingness to trade current consumption for retirement consumption. At the tangency between the *UU* and *PP* curves, point

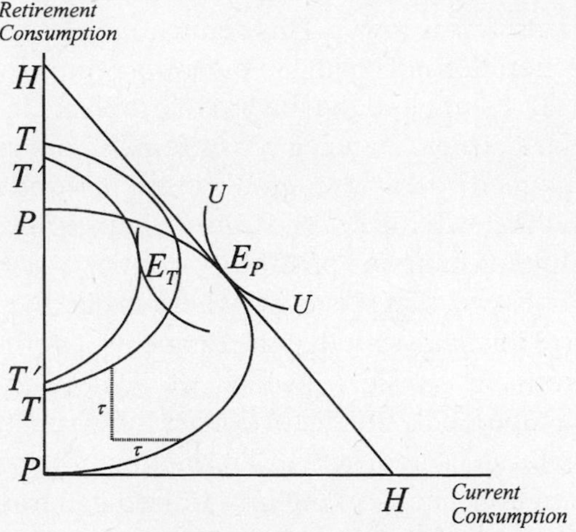

Figure 9.1 Trade-off between Current and Retirement Consumption

E_P, we have the levels of working and retirement consumption that best fits the working generation's tastes given the set of possible combinations available. Because retirement consumption is financed by the sale of capital, this point determines the capital stock that will be transferred to the next working generation.

The simplest way to show the effect of an intergeneration transfer is to use a lump sum tax to provide each member of the current working generation with a guaranteed payment during retirement. This changes the ability of the current working generation to trade current consumption for retirement consumption. On the one hand, current resources available to the working generation are reduced because of the tax, while at the same time they are guaranteed an equal amount of additional retirement consumption. In figure 9.1, we show the after-intergeneration transfer frontier as the curve *TT*, which is obtained by transforming any point on the *PP* curve by subtracting the tax, represented by τ in the figure, from current consumption and adding the tax to future consumption. The fact that interest rates are positive insures that the private system equilibrium point, E_P, is to the right of the intersection of the *PP* and *TT* curves. As a result, the intergenerational transfer best equilibrium must be inferior to that obtained without the transfer.[5]

It is also clear from the figure that total output in a world with intergenerational transfers is lower. This reduction in output results from the working generation not having to put away capital for its retirement consumption. To compound the incentive problems involved with intergenerational transfer financing of retirement, the reduction in the capital stock implied by the new equilibrium will result in an increased price of capital that will further shift the *TT* curve inward.[6] This final placement of the consumption possibility frontier we denote as *T′ T′* in figure 9.1 and observe that it is everywhere inside the *TT* curve. The striking result of this analysis is that the financing of retirement through an intergenerational transfer—even if we achieve the generational transfer with a supposedly nondistortionary lump sum tax—is a reduction in the capital stock and, hence, a reduction of goods available for consumption to both the working and retired generations. Our estimate of the increase in capital stock that would result from prefunding retirement health insurance is on the order of a 13 percent greater capital stock by the year 2030.

A Cohort-based Solution

Complete solutions to Medicare's many problems must address both the flow cost of the system and its ability to provide for future recipients. We present an approach that is based on each generation prepaying its own Medicare. Since prepaying only deals with the problem of providing for future beneficiaries of the existing Medicare program, we also design an alternative benefit package and price this package. Our alternative package, on a total-cost-to-recipient basis, is only marginally different from current Medicare; however, the incentive structure is very different. The difference in incentives has the potential of bringing the market to bear on Medicare expenditures and will result in both the buyers and sellers of health care services caring what it costs.

Medicare, as it is currently structured, provides many benefits that are not related to its primary mission of providing health care to the elderly population. However, in what follows, we restrict our discussion to the provision of health care for the elderly. Thus, we peel away all the non-age-related benefits of the current Medicare program. This is not to say that these programs are without merit, but simply that their inclusion confounds the analysis of financing health care for the elderly.[7]

In many ways providing for the health care needs of the elderly is similar to the provision of other consumption expenditures of the elderly, for example, Social Security or other retirement plans. However, there are two important differences in providing for the health care of the retired population and providing for their general living expenses. First, we have decided as a society that we will not allow differences in wealth to result in great differences in the level of health care provided for the elderly. This implicit promise of available health care upon retirement reduces the incentive for the young to provide for their own retirement health care. Second, because of rapid changes in technology, we have converted many aspects of what was at one time considered part of the normal aging process to a medical condition, thus expanding expenditures on health care. As a result, uncertainty in the level of future health care expenditures is far greater than for general living expenses.

We propose to deal with these issues by converting the financing of retirement health care to a system of prepayment by each age cohort, defined as all individuals born in a given calendar year. In this system, each worker within an age cohort will make contributions that are direct offsets to their current Medicare tax. These contributions are placed into a Private Retirement Insurance for Medical Expenditures (PRIME) account that by the time of the cohort's retirement will contain enough to pay for all retirement health care expenditures. Because of the considerable uncertainty concerning retirement health care expenditures at the time a cohort begins contributing, the level of contributions must be adjusted as a cohort ages and more information concerning future medical care needs is consequently revealed.[8]

We estimate the required PRIME account contribution rates on the basis of no survivorship benefits. In other words, we do not require that in addition to a cohort insuring against the cost of retirement health care, members of a cohort must also purchase life insurance.[9] Just as with the current Medicare program, the insurance we are proposing pays no death benefits to survivors. In its simplest form, catastrophic retirement health insurance coverage is purchased during a worker's years in the labor force. The specific insurance we are proposing is comparable to today's $2,500 deductible policies that pay all expenses above the deductible. We will also propose a movement toward long-term retirement health care contracts as one way out of the adverse selection problems inherent in current health markets.

Our estimates of the cost of converting from the existing Medicare system to one where each cohort prepays its retirement health care are based on actuarial simulations similar to those used by the Medicare Trustees. With this foundation in place, we can evaluate the cost and feasibility of the transition. Moving away from intergenerational financing of retirement health care will result in an increase in the nation's capital stock and therefore an increase in the nation's income. In the following analysis, however, we ignore this surge in income and base all our forecasts on past trends. While our forecasts are based on an actuarial model similar to that used by the Medicare Trustees, we make our own earnings forecasts to identify age cohort life-cycle earnings profiles, and we estimate the cost of an alternative benefit structure.

The long-run actuarial projections of the current Medicare system and our prepaid system rest on projections of population trends, real wage growth, and real benefit growth. With pay-as-you-go financing and stable tax rates, benefits can grow at a rate equal to the tax base growth rate. Because Medicare benefits have grown at rates that far outpace the combined growth in the labor force and real wages, the tax rate and taxable earnings levels have been increased numerous times over the program's first thirty years. The fact that all labor earnings are now subject to the Medicare payroll tax allows us to project the growth in tax receipts by simply analyzing the growth in annual earnings.[10]

The fundamental equation for the consideration of the problem of prefunding the benefit stream for new labor force entrants is that the present value of contributions made to the system during an individual's working years must be adequate to fund the present value of the retirement years benefit stream. By employing this fundamental equation, it is possible to calculate for any age cohort the contribution rate required of the representative individuals in that cohort. To calculate this required contribution rate, cohort life-cycle earnings and retirement medical benefits must be estimated. In what follows, we present our estimates of future annual earnings based on a decomposition among labor force participation, annual hours worked, real hourly wage components on the one hand, and future expected benefits on the other.

Earnings Forecast

In another work (Rettenmaier and Saving 1999), we have estimated several alternative aggregate earnings forecasts. Here we briefly describe our forecasting methods, which are based on historical growth rates for the wage, labor force participation, and hours worked components of annual earnings.

Over the last twenty years, the cross-sectional evidence indicates that the annual earnings profile for women continues to approach that for men, both for full-time, full-year workers and for the profiles that include part-time workers and nonworkers. Further, among women, cohort-based profiles tell a very different story than do cross-sectional profiles. The rise in female labor force participation, increased human capital investments, and greater labor force continuity means that cross-sectional age earnings profiles will likely underestimate younger women's real earnings and participation later in life.

We base our forecasts of earnings growth rates on data from the1964 to 1996 March Demographic Supplements to the Current Population Survey (CPS). The March Supplement questions pertain to labor market behavior during the previous year, allowing us to use data for the years from 1963 to 1995. All earnings data are converted to 1995 dollars using the Personal Consumption Expenditures implicit price deflator.[11] We adopted a technique that allowed us to track the historical changes in work participation, hours worked, and wages for different categories of workers, allowing different subsets of the labor force to experience differing growth rates for each of the earnings components.

To forecast the total tax base, and ultimately the cohort profiles required for the contribution rate estimates, we rely on the following accounting. Rather than using one-year intervals, we have identified twelve age groups—16 to 19, 20 to 24, 25 to 29, 30 to 34, 35 to 39, 40 to 44, 45 to 49, 50 to 54, 55 to 59, 60 to 64, 65 to 69, and 70 to 75—and five categories for years of education—0 to 11, 12, 13 to 15, 16, and 17+. For each of the resulting age-education cells, we have data on annual earnings, number of individuals, proportion working, and average annual hours worked and the average hourly wage, conditional on participation. With twelve age groups and five education cells for each sex, we have 116 age-by-education-by-sex cells, after omitting the cells for the youngest age group and top two education cells. For each of these cells and each of the annual earnings components, we evaluated a set of growth rate calculations. The simulations that follow are based on a growth rate that weights recent changes more heavily than changes occurring in the earlier periods.[12]

The next step in forecasting Medicare revenues is to apply the forecasted growth rates to the 1995 values for participation, hours, and real wage in each cell and predict future levels. To forecast aggregate earnings, however, we must also forecast the final component, the number of individuals in each cell. For the age distribution in future years, we have relied on the Census Bureau's intermediate population projections for 1995 to 2050. We then use the CPS data to calculate the proportion of each age group in the five education cells. The sex by age by education progression is imputed to the yet-to-be-born cohorts using a weighted average based on the baby boom generation's education attainment, excluding the first five birth cohorts.[13] From the aggregate forecast we can identify both cross-sectional and cohort age earnings profiles. For each cohort, then, we have an estimate of the path that average earnings for men and women will follow over their remaining lifetime.

Estimating the Cost of Retirement Health Care

While our emphasis is on moving toward prepaid medical insurance for the elderly, this task becomes easier if we simultaneously address the growth in per capita medical expenditures by introducing an alternative form of insurance for those cohorts who are in the prefunded system. In this section, the estimated cost of $2,500 deductible catastrophic insurance for elderly beneficiaries is presented and compared to the cost of standard Medicare benefits. The advantages of the higher-deductible policy we propose are twofold. Higher deductibles reduce the level of expenditures relative to policies with first-dollar coverage or policies with low coinsurance rates and may also affect the rate of expenditure growth. The benchmarks for the relative effects of coinsurance rates and deductibles on medical expenditures were established in the RAND Health Insurance Experiment (HIE).

We map our proposed $2,500 deductible and current Medicare into the RAND simulation model's results reported in appendix G of Keeler et al. (1988). The authors estimate the expenditures for a range of policies that are characterized by their coinsurance rate and their maximum dollar expenditures (MDE). Between 1983—the year in which the simulation model expenditures are denominated—and 1998, per capita Medicare expenditures grew by a factor of 2.94. If a $2,500 deductible, in 1998 dollars, with 100 percent coverage above the deductible was placed in the 1983 simulation model output, it would be equivalent to a policy with 100 percent coinsurance up to a MDE of $851. Such a policy is bounded by the 100 percent coinsurance/$500 MDE and the 100 percent coinsurance/$1,000 MDE policies in the RAND study. Mapping the current Medicare package into the RAND simulation results is more difficult. In short, we assume that individuals with some sort of Medigap policy or Medicaid coverage behave as if they have free care, and those with no supplement behave as if they had a policy with 25 percent coinsurance and a $1,000 (in 1983 dollars) MDE policy.

Table 9.1 presents total expenditures, Medicare benefits, and the premiums that would be necessary to purchase a high-deductible policy. The data on which the estimates are based are drawn from the Health Care Financing Administration's (HCFA) 1995 Cost and Use File. This file contains, among other things, individually based re-

Table 9.1 Total Expenditures, Medicare Benefits, and Estimated $2,500 Deductible Policy Premiums by Age, Based on the 1995 Cost and Use File Inflated to 1998 Dollars

Age Group	Total Expenditures	Medicare Benefits	$2,500 Deductible Policy Premiums
All, 65+	6,836	5,475	4,170
65–66	4,460	3,464	2,714
67–68	4,946	3,769	2,914
69–70	5,429	4,163	3,102
71–72	6,619	5,297	4,018
73–74	7,147	5,691	4,387
75–79	7,063	5,742	4,296
80–84	8,398	6,852	5,243
85+	9,596	7,871	6,022

NOTE: Total expenditures are the sum of expenditures in the following categories: home health, hospice, inpatient hospital, institutional, medical provider, and outpatient hospital. Medicare benefits are the sum of Part A and Part B reimbursements for fee-for-service patients and are equal to Medicare payments to HMOs for HMO patients.

sponses to the Medicare Current Beneficiary Survey and data from HCFA administrative records. The data provide a detailed picture of expenditures by type of event and by source of payment. We used the total expenditure, Medicare payment, and supplementary coverage indicators to calculate age-specific premium estimates. The estimated premium is the average of the expenditures above the deductible after accounting for the expenditure reduction effects associated with the high deductible.

Average Medicare benefits were $5,475 in 1998 dollars, accounting for 80 percent of an average beneficiary's total medical expenditures. Assuming no administrative costs, the Medicare benefits would represent the cost of a similarly structured private insurance policy. To compare the cost of the Medicare policy to the cost of our high-deductible policy, we net out the current Part B monthly premium of $43.80 that is paid by beneficiaries. This results in a net Medicare benefit of $4,949, which is only 19 percent higher than the estimated price of our high-deductible policy.

Even without prefunding, one of the recurring reform proposals is to allow private insurers to compete in the Medicare fee-for-service market. However, the theoretical problems confronting insurance markets—adverse selection and moral hazard—are well-known, as are some of their manifestations, such as the "death spiral" of generous plans, as relatively low-cost individuals leave the pool in successive rounds of defections, until those remaining are too few, and too costly, to profitably insure. These problems have historically been the stumbling block for broad proposals that include the participation of private insurers in the Medicare market.

These problems are manifested by the difficulty workers face in continuing employment-based coverage after leaving a job, or similarly, the transferability of employment-based coverage. Problems arise largely because insurance contracts are short term so that if a policyholder gets a long-term illness that may affect job status, the current insurer has every incentive to drop coverage at the end of the period. Likewise, other potential insurers would lose money if they offered insurance to an ill person at the same premium as a healthy person, and so seek to avoid those with preexisting conditions.

It is tempting to simply obligate the current insurer to offer continued coverage at the same rate. However, this ties the relatively sick to one insurer; moreover, the same restrictions must be placed on the relatively healthy, who have an incentive to switch insurers for cheaper rates, leaving the original insurer with the "lemons." Tying consumers to one insurer, however, is inimical to competition. Because we have prepaid our retirement health care, everyone at any predetermined retirement age—65, for example—has the purchasing power to buy a lifetime health care contract. Such lifetime contracts, properly structured, can overcome some or all of the adverse selection problems of single-year contracts and allow consumers complete choice as to who provides their health care.

An institution that can accomplish this outcome is the institution of a market for risk categories of recipients. Each participating provider prices lifetime care for each age and risk category. At times specified in the contract—perhaps the end of each year—any participant can leave a provider, and the provider must pay the recipient the present value of that participant's expected future health care benefits. This payment must be the same amount that the provider charges new participants of the same age and health status. Thus, providers are indifferent between a participant staying or leaving, and, moreover, participants can move to other providers at will.[14]

Once the initial purchase of retirement health insurance is accomplished, insurance companies can charge actuarially fair individual premiums in the spot market. Basically, the plan involves individually priced, actuarially fair health insurance combined with what is in effect premium insurance. This plan, as it allows complete individual mobility, encourages competition among insurers, which encourages quality, variety, and innovation.

While the feasibility of such a plan in practice has yet to be demonstrated, long-term retirement health contracts offer a way out of the principal difficulties that result from one-sided one-year contracts currently in use. Current insurance markets suffer from adverse selection problems to a greater extent than necessary because insurers are not permitted to set premiums on the basis of observable information such as health history. Thus, although cost-relevant information is available, it is not used by insurers; so the situation is as if there were asymmetric information. For long-term contracts, such asymmetric information is less important since it usually involves near-term outcomes. Furthermore, the equity issues concerning the use of all cost-relevant information become moot because once individuals are in the system, their funds are always available to transfer to any other carrier.

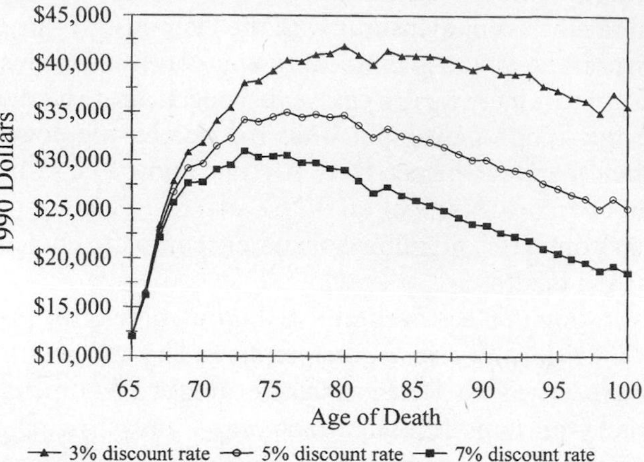

Figure 9.2 Present Value at Age 65 of Medicare Payment, by Age of Death
The present values in the figure above are based on the benefit profiles by age of death presented in a paper by James Lubitz, James Beebe, and Colin Baker, "Longevity and Medicare Expenditures," *New England Journal of Medicine* (April 1995): 999–1,003.

The implementation of long-term insurance with free choice is easier for retirees with prepaid health care than for those of working age. First, because it is prefunded, there is not the problem of people spending their severance payments or not being able to pay amounts due their current insurer. A switch from one insurer to another can be effected by the original insurer simply by paying the new insurer the present value of remaining expected lifetime health care costs.

Furthermore, adverse selection problems and screening on the part of insurers at the beginning are substantially mitigated by the long-term nature of the obligations of the contract. In figure 9.2, the present value of average retirement health care costs by age of death, for three discount rates, is presented. For any discount rate, the present value of expenses are lower for those who die soon after retirement and quite similar for all those who reach 70 years of age. Thus, in a present value sense, health status involves two offsetting effects on expected health expenses. Those currently healthy live longer and therefore incur more minor expenses, while those who are obviously in poor health, whose immediate expenses are higher, are likely to die relatively soon, and thus have lower total retirement health expenses. As a result, long-term health care contracts have the property that those who are obviously ill and in need of care are not the ones insurers seek to avoid. If anything the sickest are the most profitable and should be welcomed by insurers. Furthermore, when people enter the system, it is the distribution of the present value of medical expenditures that concerns insurers, not the distribution of expenditures in the cross section. The former distribution is less skewed than the latter. Because the typical screening techniques employed by insurers are less effective in partitioning beneficiaries between low and high costs, insurers will start off with a distribution much closer to a random draw.

Contribution Rate Estimates

The earnings forecasts and the two age-specific benefit vectors combined with mortality rates for each living cohort allow us to calculate the required contribution rate under several rate-of-return and growth rate assumptions. The mortality estimates we use are based on predicted life expectancies from the Census Bureau's middle series. The 1995, 2005, and 2050 life tables are used along with linear interpolations by age for the intervening years and for the years beyond 2050.

In table 9.2, we show estimates of required contribution rates for

Table 9.2 Required Annual Contributions Beginning at Age 22 as a Percent of Life-Cycle Earnings

Rate of Return	Growth Rate in Per Capita Medical Expenditures	Medicare Replacement	$2,500 Deductible Policy
5.4	1	2.19	1.85
5.4	2	3.77	3.19
5.4	HCFA	2.87	2.43
6.4	1	1.52	1.29
6.4	2	2.61	2.21
6.4	HCFA	1.99	1.69
9.0	1	0.59	0.51
9.0	2	1.00	0.85
9.0	HCFA	0.78	0.66

NOTE: The HCFA growth rate in per capita medical expenditures is based on the approximated growth rates assumed in the 1998 Trustees Report. For years 1998 to 2002, the growth rate is 1 percent; from 2003 to 2010, it is 3.5 percent; for the years 2011 to 2022, it declines at a constant rate to 0.9 percent—the trustees' ultimate real wage growth assumption—and remains at 0.9 percent in all subsequent years.

new labor force entrants, assumed to enter the labor force at 22 years of age, for combinations of three rates of return, three rates of growth in retirement health care expenditures, and two benefit configurations.

Rates of Return

First, Feldstein and Samwick (1997) estimate that a portfolio "of 60 percent equity and 40 percent debt had a yield of about 5.4 percent over both the postwar period and the period since1926." Second, our estimates of the real rate of return on the Standard and Poors 500, including dividend reinvestment for the last sixty years, is 6.4 percent. Finally, Feldstein and Samwick argue that if corporate taxes at all levels take 40 percent of pretax debt and equity income, then a 5.4 percent after-tax return is equivalent to a 9 percent pretax return.

Expenditure Growth Rates

The contribution rates presented in table 9.2 are based on three alternative rates of growth of per capita health care expenditures scenarios. The first two are simple fixed real growth rates in health care expenditures, 1 and 2 percent, applied to all future periods. The third real health care growth rate assumption considered is the growth rate pattern used in the 1998 Medicare Trustees Report. The trustees assume for the years 1998 to 2002 a real per capita growth rate of 1 percent, followed by real per capita growth of 3.5 percent for the years 2003 to 2010; and they assume that real per capita growth of health care expenditures will fall to 0.9 percent by 2022, then remain at this level for the remainder of the time considered.

Benefit Configuration

Our contribution rate estimates are calculated for two alternative benefit configurations. First, we calculate the cost of prepaying for the existing Medicare benefits net of premiums but allowing the benefits to grow at the rates of growth discussed above. Second, we construct the cost of providing a $2,500 deductible health care policy that covers all expenditures once the deductible is met. Since this latter benefit structure does not have first-dollar coverage, it has the potential of affecting the level of health care expenditures.

As the estimates in table 9.2 indicate, the contribution rate for entering cohorts ranges from a low of 0.51 percent to a high of 3.77 percent. In 1998, Medicare's total expenditures associated with treating the population 65 and above, net of premium payments, represented an amount that would be equal to 4.24 percent of taxable payroll. Thus, for all per capita health care expenditure growth rates and rates-of-return assumptions, the contribution rate is less than the implied tax rate. Moreover, the majority of the contribution rates are less than the stated 2.9 percent Hospitalization Insurance tax rate.

Transition Cost Estimates

In the following estimates of the cost of the transition to our privatized system, we restrict ourselves to the assumption of a 5.4 percent rate of return. This rate of return is the after-tax rate on a balanced portfolio, which we combine with our two medical care expenditure growth rates and the Medicare growth rates used by HCFA. A final consideration is whether or not the $2,500 deductible insurance plan will affect the level of health care usage, for which there is considerable evidence, and stem the growth in medical care expenditures. We would expect such policies to spur cost-reducing innovations in the production of services that fall below the deductible as suppliers compete for the significant quantity of first dollars. However, for purposes of our transition cost estimates, we have assumed that moving to a no-first-dollar coverage world has no effect on the growth in health care expenditures, and we treat the growth rate as an input in our simulations.

During the transition to a cohort-based financing system, the health care costs of the currently retired population and those close to the retirement age must be paid at the same time that contributions to cohort accounts are being made. As the contribution rates presented in table 9.2 indicate, the new insurance can be purchased over younger cohorts' lives at rates that are less than the current implied full Medicare tax rate of 4.24 percent, and in most cases at rates even less than the dedicated tax of 2.9 percent of payroll. Therefore, during a shift to cohort-based financing, it is possible to offset part of the transition cost with the difference between the full tax rate and the cohort contribution rate. Figure 9.3 illustrates the expected revenues and expenditures under the status quo and under the assumption of an immediate transition to cohort-based financing.

The series presented in figure 9.3 were calculated based on the as-

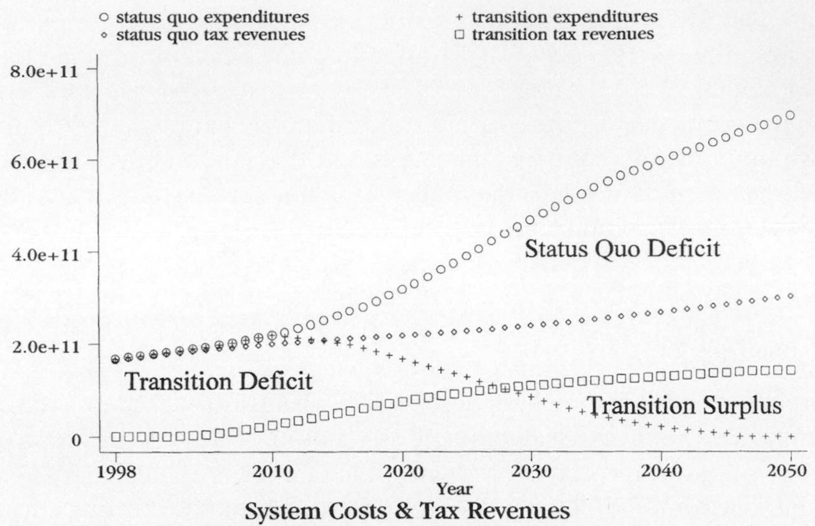

Figure 9.3 System Costs and Tax Revenues

sumptions that the real rate of return is 5.4 percent and the growth rate in per capita medical expenditures is 1 percent. Individuals in the prefunded system are assumed to buy a benefit vector that is equal in value to the current Medicare package net of premium. Further, the implied tax rate of 4.24 percent is assumed to remain in effect until 2080. The series identified as the status quo expenditures is equal to real Medicare benefits, net of premium payments, growing at 1 percent per year for the population 65 and above. The status quo tax revenues are equal to 4.24 percent of aggregate labor earnings. The present value of the difference between these series is the status quo unfunded liability.

The other two series in figure 9.3 reflect the expenditures and revenues associated with a transition to prefunded cohort-based retirement health insurance. For our purposes we place all individuals born in 1946 or later into the new system (shifting all the baby boomers to the new system). With this design, transition expenditures are equal to status quo expenditures out to the year 2010 (when the first of the baby boomers reach age 65). In 2011 and beyond, no new beneficiaries are added to the old system, and consequently transition expenditures continuously decline after 2010 and approach zero by 2046. We identify the path of the funds available to pay for the obligations that remain under the old system as the transition tax revenues.

These revenues are equal to the difference between the implied tax rate and the contribution rate times taxable earnings. For new labor force entrants, this percentage difference is 4.24 percent minus 2.19 percent, or 2.05 percent. Thus, 2.05 percent of the new labor force entrants' earnings can be used to retire the Medicare liability of those who are 52 and above in 1998. Cohorts up to the age of 39 can fund their own current Medicare equivalent retirement medical insurance for less than 4.24 percent of their remaining lifetime earnings, while cohorts up to the age of 42 can prefund the $2,500 deductible policy. Thus, for cohorts between 22 and 39 years of age in 1998, a declining portion of their earnings can be used to retire the old system's liability. Contributions to the cohort-based insurance for individuals between 40 and 51, which are in excess of the 4.24 percent implied tax, are counted against the transition tax revenues, but all of the tax revenues collected from the population 52 and above are counted as transition tax revenues. Because individuals between 40 and 52 are also placed in the prefunded system, transition tax revenues are essentially zero in 1998. The labeled areas in the graph indicate the deficits and surpluses if the status quo is maintained or if a transition to a prefunded system is made.

In table 9.3, we present the present value under the current tax burden of the unfunded liability associated with three scenarios: the status quo (the current Medicare benefit and tax structure), a prefunded version of current Medicare benefits, and the prefunding of the $2,500 deductible Medicare substitute described above. The prefunded results all assume a real rate of return on PRIME account investments equal to 5.4 percent.

Table 9.3 Present Value of Unfunded Liabilities: Current System and 1998 Transition to a Prefunded System ($Billions 1998 Dollars)

			Transition	
Rate of Return	**Growth Rate in Per Capita Medical Expenditures**	**Status Quo**	**Medicare Replacement**	**$2,500 Deductible Policy**
5.4	1	5,566	1,640	841
5.4	2	11,674	5,264	3,992
5.4	HCFA	9,270	4,112	3,059

NOTE: The rate of return on government bonds used to calculate the present values is 2.8 percent—the rate used in the 1998 Medicare Trustees report. The last year in the simulation is 2080.

The most striking result is that maintaining the status quo is significantly more costly than switching to a prefunded system, even one that keeps the current Medicare benefit structure intact. The present value of the status quo unfunded liability ranges from \$5.6 trillion, assuming a constant 1 percent growth in real Medicare benefits, to \$11.6 trillion based on a constant 2 percent growth in real Medicare benefits. The present value of the unfunded liability of prefunding current Medicare benefits ranges from \$1.6 trillion to \$5.2 trillion (or, 30 percent and 45 percent of the cost of maintaining the status quo). Prefunding our high-deductible Medicare implies present values of unfunded liabilities ranging from \$0.8 trillion to \$4.0 trillion (or, 15 percent and 34 percent of the cost of maintaining the status quo). If we adopt HCFA's growth rate assumptions, the transition cost in which a package equal in value to Medicare is purchased by those in the prefunded system can be accomplished for 44 percent of the cost of maintaining the status quo. Under these conditions, prefunding the no-first-dollar Medicare plan can be accomplished for less that one-third the cost of the status quo.

Since any solution to the Medicare financing crisis must involve an increase in taxes, in table 9.4 we present the additional tax rates—over and above the full implied tax rate of 4.24 percent—that would be necessary to pay off the unfunded liability attributed to each alternative.[15] For example, if the growth rate in per capita medical expenditures is assumed to be 1 percent (the first row in table 9.4), then to maintain the status quo, the tax rate necessary to make the system solvent would be 7.30 percent (4.24 + 3.06). Paying off the transition completely under the same set of assumptions but using prefunding to pay for the current level of Medicare benefits would require a tax hike of only 0.9 percentage points, or a total tax rate of 5.14 percent. Finally, prepaying for no-first-dollar coverage, \$2,500 deductible Medicare would require an immediate increase in the tax rate of only 0.46 percentage points, or a total tax rate of 4.70 percent.

Using the results reported in table 9.4, the transition to prepayment would work as follows: The Medicare tax rate is raised immediately to 5.14 percent or 4.70 percent, depending on whether we retain current Medicare or move to no-first-dollar Medicare. These tax rates are a full 2.16 or 2.60 percentage points lower than would be necessary to take care of the status quo debt. The additional tax revenues collected from this extra tax are added to the transition tax revenues and the difference between the new total revenue and the transition cost is covered

Table 9.4 Additional Taxes: Current System Remains Intact and 1998 Transition to a Prefunded System (Percentage Points)

			Transition	
Rate of Return	**Growth Rate in Per Capita Medical Expenditures**	**Status Quo**	**Medicare Replacement**	**$2,500 Deductible Policy**
5.4	1	3.06	0.90	0.46
5.4	2	6.41	2.89	2.19
5.4	HCFA	5.09	2.26	1.68

NOTE: The rate of return on government bonds used to calculate the present values is 2.8 percent—the rate used in the 1998 Medicare Trustees report. The last year in the simulation is 2080.

by additional temporary government borrowing, to be paid off when the financing surplus occurs. Recall from figure 9.2 that the transition revenues begin to exceed costs and are used to pay off the borrowed funds within thirty years, even before any additional tax revenues are added. Thus, the earmarked Medicare debt will begin to be paid off well before thirty years, and a total payoff will occur in 2080.[16]

While tables 9.3 and 9.4 are instructive in revealing the benefits of moving to prepaid financing of Medicare, they fail to reveal the whole picture. In comparing the status quo with prepaid financing, we have ignored the impact of generational transfers on the nation's capital stock. Since we estimate that the nation's net capital stock will rise 13 percent by 2030 as the additional government borrowing is offset by the aggregate funds accumulated in the PRIME accounts, national income will be higher than that assumed in the above estimates of the required tax rates. Therefore, the tax rates required to fund the transition to prepaid financing of Medicare are overestimated, and both tables 9.3 and 9.4 underestimate the benefits of moving to a prepaid cohort-based system of financing Medicare.

Conclusion

Converting the current pay-as-you-go system of financing Medicare to a cohort-based system can be accomplished if prompt action is taken. Both Parts A and B of Medicare can be replaced with fully funded cohort-based real investment. Such investment will increase the nation's capital stock and provide the resources necessary to fund the retirement medical care of the baby boomers, while at the same time protecting the rights of older generations to retirement medical care.

The problem of the retirement population surge that will occur as the baby boomers leave the labor force is compounded by the fact that real per capita health care expenditures have been rising faster for the Medicare population than for the population as a whole. Our ability to cope with the unfunded Medicare liability depends on our willingness to get control of these out-of-control health care expenditures by the Medicare-covered populations. The approach we have suggested is the conversion of the current Parts A and B of Medicare into health insurance consisting of a high deductible and then 100 percent coverage. This type of health coverage makes consumers care what health care costs and will play a major role in restoring competition to the industry.

Our estimates indicate that a transition to prefunded Medicare can be accomplished at a cost that is considerably less than the cost of maintaining pay-as-you-go financing. The transition would be designed such that all individuals born in 1946 and later would be switched to prefunded insurance. Because cohorts 42 years of age and younger in 1998 can purchase the proposed insurance at rates that are less than the implied Medicare tax of 4.24 percent, their excess contributions can go toward funding the older cohorts, those born before 1946, who remain in the to-be-amended Medicare system. The younger cohorts' contributions will also be used to prefund part of the insurance of the group between 43 and 52 years of age. We estimate that the transition will save the country money—when compared to maintaining the status quo. Once the last of the over-52 group has left the system, all future generations are self-funded. Thus, a population surge will not produce a financing bind again.

When one considers the large difference in the potential unfunded liability of the current system and our cohort-based alternative, one wonders, Where is the free lunch? After a thorough look at our proposal, however, it will be clear that there is no free lunch, but there is a considerably cheaper lunch that is of better quality than the one we are currently committed to buying. The current generational transfer system of financing Medicare reduces the nation's capital stock and thereby reduces national income. By moving to prepaid financing, we remove the disincentives to invest and the nation experiences an increase in capital and income. It is this increase in capital that provides the additional resources available to pay off most, but not all, of the current system's unfunded liability. Moving to prepaid retirement health insurance is just good business.

Even if it is good business to switch to cohort-based financing, why is it so important to do it now? The answer lies in the income-generating power of the baby boom generation. While the pending retirement of the baby boomers looms like a dark cloud over the present Medicare system, these same baby boomers can save the system if we can harness their earning power. But to do this we must act quickly. We must move all the baby boomers into the new system.

Notes

1. The trend is for all areas of medical care to have increased third-party participation so that years are being taken out of the "who cares what it costs" loop. For example, between 1990 and 1997 the cost of prescription drugs paid out-of-pocket dropped from 48 to 29 percent and, as expected, real per capita expenditures grew 59 percent.

2. See A. W. Wilcox (1936) for a complete discussion of the act and the public finance aspects of the Old-Age Reserve Account, now referred to as the Social Security Trust Fund.

3. If the trust fund buys back some of your outstanding debt rather than using it to support your current consumption, then the result is exactly the same as buying bonds from others because the proceeds in the trust fund represent a net addition to your asset position and are, therefore, available for use later. If, on the other hand, you simply issue bonds to the trust fund and spend the proceeds on current consumption, your net asset position deteriorates and there are no funds available for use later.

4. An excellent review of the history of Medicare provisions is contained in the annual statistical supplement to the 1996 *Social Security Bulletin*.

5. The only way the original equilibrium can be to the left of the intersection of the *TT* and *PP* curves is for individuals to strongly prefer consumption in their retirement years to current consumption, that is, to strongly prefer the future. Such preferences for the future would imply negative interest rates, which is contradicted by reality.

6. The price of capital must equal the marginal productivity of capital, which is inversely related to the capital stock. For a complete discussion of this relation see Rettenmaier and Saving (1999), chapter 3.

7. Thus, transfers to the poor are not considered because being poor is not age related. In a sense, all poor should be treated by the system in a similar manner, independent of age.

8. An additional benefit of cohort-based financing is that it eliminates cohort size risk of the form we are now facing with the pending retirement of the baby boom generation. If the population age distribution experiences a bulge because of larger-than-normal fertility or immigration, the contribution to retirement medical insurance of these cohorts will rise, maintaining the same per capita value as smaller cohorts.

9. Tying a mandatory life insurance program to the purchase of retirement medical insurance simply increases the cost. In addition, we already have a mandatory life insurance program contained in Social Security.

10. Only the Hospitalization Insurance portion of Medicare has a dedicated payroll tax. In 1994 the maximum earnings subject to the tax was raised from $135,000 to its current unlimited level.

11. Annual earnings were defined as the sum of wage and salary and self-employment income. Top coded wages were inflated by a factor of 1.5 and top coded self-employment income by a factor of 2. Individuals younger than 16 and those older than 75 were excluded.

12. For a complete description of how earnings were forecasted, see Rettenmaier and Saving (1999). The growth rates we compared are drawn from those presented in Murphy and Welch (1992).

13. The birth cohorts 1946 to 1950 were excluded to omit the possible upward bias in male educational attainment during the Vietnam War. Educational attainment of the younger baby boom cohorts is weighted more heavily and is imputed to current cohorts younger than 24 years of age. For older current cohorts the empirical distribution is used.

14. This solution is a variant of one analyzed by John H. Cochrane in "Time-Consistent Health Insurance," *Journal of Political Economy* 103 (June 1995): 445–73. Cochrane's plan, in the context of nonretirees, works along the following lines: Specifics may vary but the key feature is a severance payment. In the beginning, nothing is known about individual-level expected health expenses. Individuals buy into health insurance at a premium that reflects average expenses, but over time individuals will suffer health shocks. As part of the insurance contract, at the end of each period insurers pay to each less healthy individual a severance payment equal to the present value of the increase in expected future costs. In this way, the ill individual can then afford to buy actuarially fair spot insurance, while paying out-of-pocket only the average premium. Conversely, if an individual becomes healthier than average, they must pay their insurer an amount equal to the reduction in expected costs. This covers, on average, the severance payments to those becoming less healthy.

15. It should be noted that because the simulation is terminated in 2080, the status quo unfunded liability is underestimated because in that year and beyond, the status quo expenditures exceed the status quo revenues. In contrast, the transition expenditures decline to zero as the individuals in the old system die.

16. It is important to bear in mind that if the present pay-as-you-go system of financing Medicare is retained, even with the increase in the tax rate suggested in table 9.4, the system will be in deficit forever because the tax rate presented only makes the system solvent out to the year 2080.

References

Board of Trustees of the Federal Hospital Insurance Trust Fund. 1998. *1998 Annual Report of the Board of Trustees of the Federal Hospital Insurance Trust Fund*. Washington, D.C.

Board of Trustees of the Federal Supplementary Medical Insurance Trust Fund. 1998. *1998 Annual Report of the Board of Trustees of the Federal Supplementary Medical Insurance Trust Fund* (April). Washington, D.C.

Feldstein, Martin. 1996. "The Missing Piece in Policy Analysis: Social Security Reform." Richard T. Ely Lecture. *The American Economic Review* 86 (no. 2, May): 1–14.

Feldstein, Martin, and Andrew A. Samwick. 1997. "The Economics of Prefunding Social Security and Medicare Benefits." NBER Working Paper 6055.

Keeler, Emmett B., Joan L. Buchanan, John E. Rolph, Janet M. Hanley, and David M. Reboussin. 1988. "The Demand for Episodes of Medical Treatment in the Health Insurance Experiment" (March). RAND Health Insurance Experiment Series.

Murphy, Kevin M., and Finis Welch. 1992. "Real Wages 1963–1990." Santa Monica, Calif.: Unicon Research Corporation.

Rettenmaier, Andrew J., and Thomas R. Saving. 1999. *The Economics of Medicare Reform*. Forthcoming. The Upjohn Institute.

Social Security Administration. 1996. *Social Security Bulletin Annual Statistical Supplement*. Washington, D.C.: U.S. Government Printing Office.

Thompson, Lawrence H. 1983. "The Social Security Reform Debate." *Journal of Economic Literature* XXI (no. 4, December): 1,425–67.

Willcox, A. W. 1937. "The Old-Age Reserve Account—A Problem in Government Finance." *The Quarterly Journal of Economics* 51: 444–48.

Contributors

Henry J. Aaron
The Brookings Institution
1775 Massachusetts Ave. NW
Washington, DC 20036
202-797-6128 (ofc.)
202-797-9181 (fax)
haaron@brook.edu

David M. Cutler
Harvard University
Department of Economics
Cambridge, MA 02138
617-496-5216 (ofc.)
617-868-2742 (fax)
dcutler@fas.harvard.edu

Victor R. Fuchs
National Bureau of Economic Research
30 Alta Road
Stanford, CA 94305
650-326-7639 (ofc.)
650-328-4163 (fax)

Jagadeesh Gokhale
Federal Reserve Bank of Cleveland
Research Department
1455 East 6th Street
Cleveland, OH 44114
216-579-2970 (ofc.)
jagadeesh.j.gokhale@clev.frb.org

Laurence J. Kotlikoff
Department of Economics
Boston University
270 Bay State Road
Boston, MA 02215
617-353-4002 (ofc.)
617-353-4001 (fax)
kotlikof@bu.edu

Marilyn Moon
Urban Institute
2100 M. Street NW
Washington, DC, 20037
202-261-5691 (ofc.)
202-223-1149 (fax)

Kevin M. Murphy
University of Chicago
Graduate School of Business
1101 East 58th Street
Chicago, IL 60637
773-702-7280 (ofc.)
773-702-2699 (fax)
kjmurphy@gsb.uchicago.edu

Mark V. Pauly
Department of Health Care Systems
University of Pennsylvania
3641 Locust Walk Center
Philadelphia, PA 19104-6218
215-898-5411 (ofc.)
215-575-7025 (fax)
pauly@wharton.upenn.edu

Andrew J. Rettenmaier
Texas A&M University
Private Enterprise Research Center
3028 Academic Building West
College Station, TX 77843-4231
409-845-7559 (ofc.)
409-845-6636 (fax)
a-rettenmaier@tamu.edu

Thomas R. Saving
Texas A&M University
Private Enterprise Research Center
3028 Academic Building West
College Station, TX 77843-4231
409-845-7559 (ofc.)
409-845-6636 (fax)
t-saving@tamu.edu

Frank Sloan
Duke University
Center for Health Policy, Law and Management
Box 90253, 125 Old Chemistry Bldg.
Durham, NC 27708
919-684-8047 (ofc.)
919-684-6246 (fax)
sloan003@mc.duke.edu

Donald H. Taylor Jr.
Duke University
Center for Health Policy, Law and Management
Box 90253, 125 Old Chemistry Bldg.
Durham, NC 27708
919-684-2361 (ofc.)
919-684-6246 (fax)
dtaylor@hpolicy.duke.edu

Index

Abbreviations are used after the page number to indicate figure (*f*), table (*t*), or endnote (*n*).